HEALTH

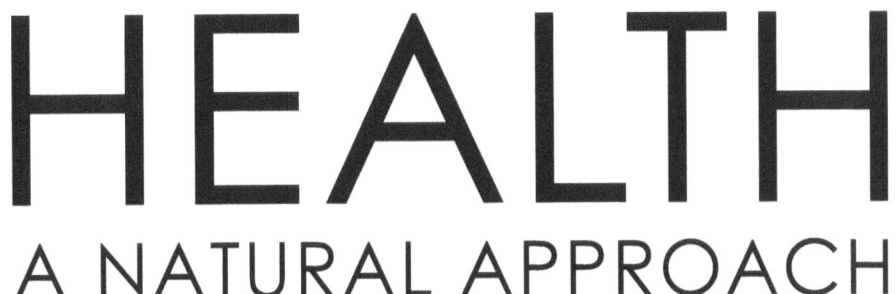

A NATURAL APPROACH

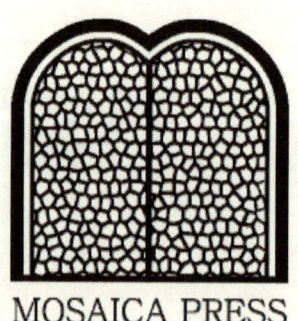

MOSAICA PRESS

HEALTH

A NATURAL APPROACH

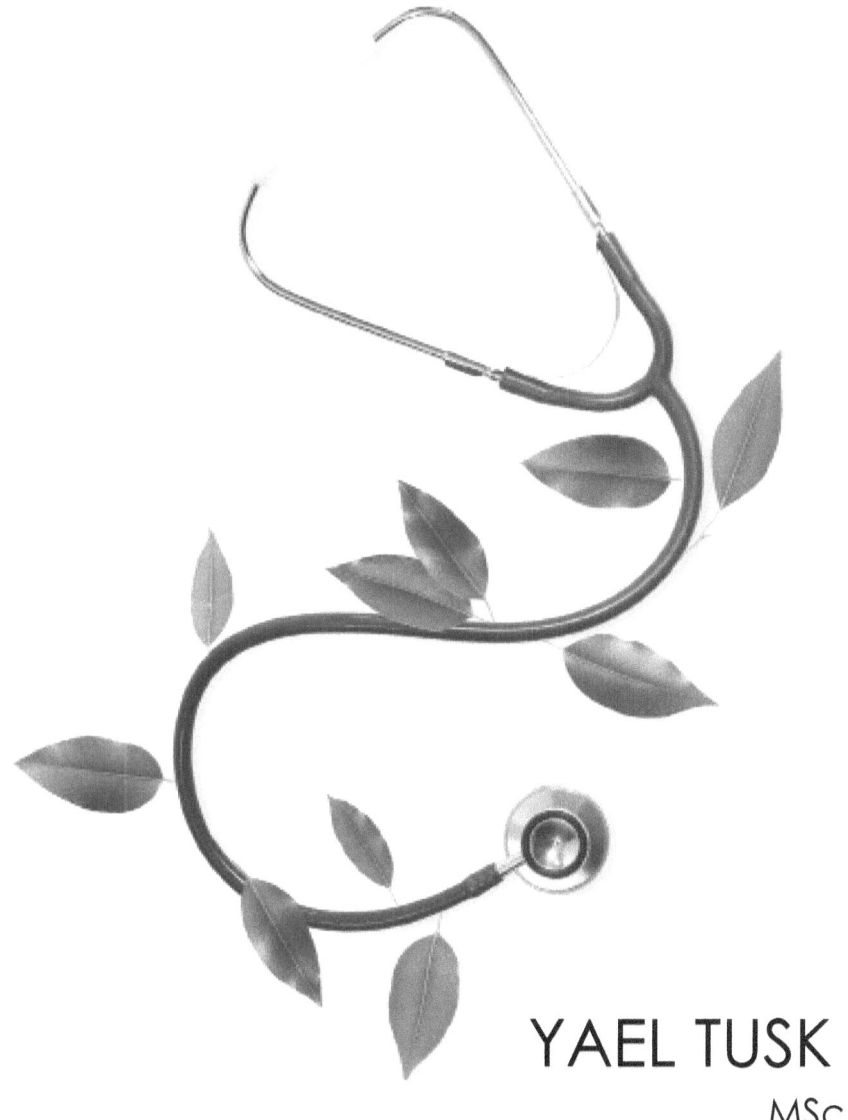

YAEL TUSK

MSc

Disclaimer: The information in this book is for educational purposes only and is not intended to replace a relationship with a healthcare provider.

TABLE OF CONTENTS

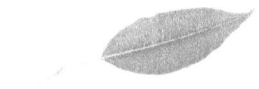

ACKNOWLEDGMENTS

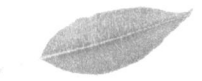

I would like to thank all of **my readers** who, with their constructive feedback and their avid interest in my columns, have encouraged me to keep researching and writing. I would also like to express my thanks to all of **my patients** who have passed through our clinic over the past decade. As we worked to improve their health, they have taught me so much. My patients have been a fount of information and inspiration.

As I was preparing this manuscript for publication, I came across a book that was published by **Mosaica Press**. I was impressed with the beautiful presentation and excellent editing. I was also pleasantly surprised to see that the book was not overly censored. This gave the impression that the publisher trusts its readers enough to allow them to see the whole story and judge for themselves. I knew that Mosaica was the address for my manuscript. Working with Mosaica has been an incredibly positive experience and I have only gratitude!

I am particularly grateful to **Varda Branfman**, editor of *The English Update*, who utilized her media outlet to help health consumers become informed. Varda was open-minded enough to publish even my most revolutionary articles, and never nixed an idea I presented to her. If she was unfamiliar with the subject matter, she went and verified it for herself, and ultimately always stood by my research. It was Varda who first encouraged me to turn my writing into a book.

I have tremendous appreciation for **my mother, Channah Trencher,** who has not only helped me with actual research, but has also helped perfect nearly every article I've written before it was published. Additionally, she has always acted as the ultimate role model for healthy skepticism in all areas of health. Her open-mindedness and willingness to learn new things and make major changes even late in the game, when most people are stuck in their ways, has been a huge inspiration for me.

Finally, I would like to express my deep gratitude to **my husband, Yoni,** who has been my foremost advocate and the perfect partner in crime. In his humility, most people do not realize that Yoni has become an expert in many areas of health, having studied our entire health library and beyond. Yoni has been my number one fan, and his support has been so complete that I hardly feel the need for anyone else's.

Special thanks to all of the generous sponsors whose contributions have helped make this book a reality. Including but not limited to: Donny and Chaya Becker, Ben and Chaya Blumenfeld, Ezzy and Chavi Dicker, Mrs. Celia Feder, Daniel and Shifra Gewurtz, Chaim and Esti Kowalsky, David and Chaya Sorah Kraus, Mrs. Gina Singer, Moish and Sandy Trencher, Yitzchok and Channah Trencher, Mrs. Fay Tusk, David and Riva Tusk, Moshe and Debbie Weiss, Shaindy and Shimshon Weiss, and Shia and Edith Zeitman. Thanks to everyone else who donated during our book campaign or preordered a sponsor's copy. We hope that you will utilize this book in good health!

Some of the material in this book was first published in *The English Update, Hamodia,* and *Tachlis Magazine* and on Arutz Sheva media network.

INTRODUCTION

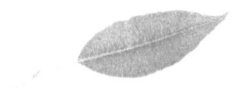

In Chinese medical school, I learned very quickly what it feels like to be the underdog. The more I studied, the more I wondered how a system as brilliant and comprehensive as Chinese medicine had been relegated to the back burner. Although our training was incredibly rigorous, I discovered that acupuncturists are not viewed with the same awe-inspiring status as doctors in the Western world, though I dare say that many doctors of Chinese medicine treat and cure a whole lot of illness and help restore health for many people.

As a holistic healthcare provider working with a medical paradigm that is brilliant, subtle, and incredibly gentle, I have learned to trust in the human body, to trust my patients' intuition, and ultimately and most importantly, to trust the Creator. Although Chinese medicine is very effective, in reality, every holistic system gently encourages the body to heal *itself*.

DO YOU BELIEVE?

When I first entered graduate school, I have to admit that I was more than a little bit wary. "What if Chinese medicine is just a bunch of baloney?" I asked myself. I was completely skeptical, but as open-minded as was possible for me at the time. I certainly *wanted* Chinese medicine to be legitimate, or I wouldn't have been there. I just couldn't help but doubt that it could actually work. Could anything besides modern medicine really work? It just didn't seem possible.

I was forced to take a leap of faith when I entered Chinese medical school, but that was the last leap of faith I took. From then on, it was experiencing the effectiveness and understanding the logic of a medical system that simply made sense that sold me. However, for over fifteen years I have been constantly asked the following question, "Do you believe in Chinese medicine?" At first, the question confused me greatly, and I had no answer. As I saw it (and still see it), if it works, then there is no need for belief, and if it doesn't work, then only a fool would believe.

There is a widely held belief that the scientific method is nearly infallible. This is very far from the truth. In fact, the way most studies are conducted, the findings and conclusions are merely a consensus of the *opinion* of the researchers who performed the study. A study's findings depend heavily on how the study was designed and what criteria were measured, all factors that are subject to biases. And expert opinion is just that. Opinion. Even widely held consensus of experts does not shape **reality**. Scientific exploration and medical research can be highly subjective, and will always be susceptible to human error, just like everything else produced my mankind. Science is the work of the human mind. It can be truly brilliant at times, but it can also be abysmally wrong at other times.

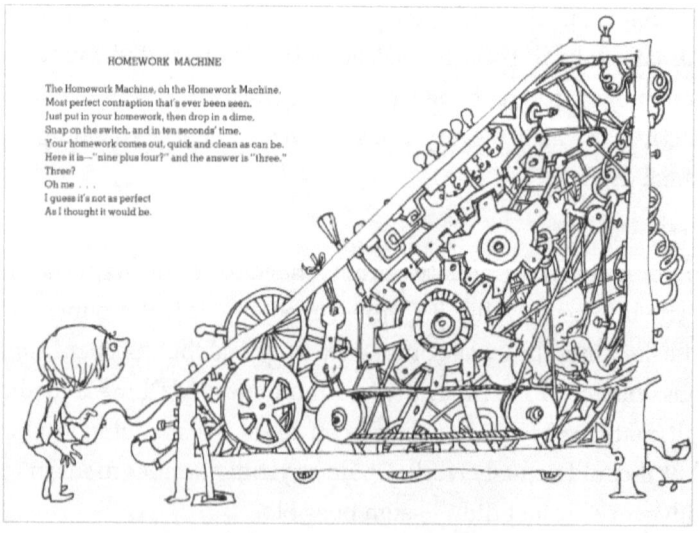

There is nothing wrong with human error — everybody makes mistakes. The problem arises when belief in science becomes an article of faith. **Faith has no place in the world of science or medicine**.

WHY BELIEF?

Why do so many people ask questions about belief? Because we have been taught to "believe" in medicine. Of course, this belief only applies to *modern* medicine. In fact, all other medical systems have been discredited by the medical establishment under the pretense of being unscientific, i.e., not "evidence based" via the scientific method. This leads to the perception that before the scientific method was developed, it was **impossible** to properly come to a valid conclusion. Hence, by default all medical systems developed outside the framework of the scientific method become "unscientific" and therefore invalid.

Modern science asserts that it is the only "evidence-based" system in existence, while *all* other systems are deemed baseless and therefore could only be "faith based." Incredibly, by asserting that evidence-based medicine and the scientific method are the epitome of scientific perfection — the ultimate truth — it becomes necessary to have *faith* in *science*, lest you be accused, heaven-forefend, of being "anti-science!"

Did you catch the unbelievable irony here? If not, let's just go over this one more time. In recent years some very passionate and scientifically minded people have started accusing whoever they feel does not have the proper *faith* in science, of being...anti-science. But if science is supposed to be flawlessly evidence based, then what place is there for belief? And what difference does it make whether someone else *believes* what you *know* to be certain truth?

There is no need to take a leap of faith with regard to one's health, when we have access to evidence and experience. Therefore, I do *not* believe in Chinese medicine, or any other medical system. I *know* from experience that Chinese medicine works well and that it's safe. I also know that it makes a lot of sense. It's logical and simple, yet brilliant. I like Chinese medicine, but that's not what this book is about. This book is about using your head.

When it comes to health, an educated decision will always serve us better than a decision based on faith. Chinese medicine is eons ahead of modern medicine, in experience and in depth of understanding health, and will always remain so; after all, they had a two-thousand-year head start, with or without the scientific method. Two thousand years of experience is certainly enough to make faith unnecessary.

HAS YOUR DOCTOR EARNED YOUR TRUST?

We've been taught to trust the experts with a nearly blind faith; to defer to their judgment. After all, they've spent so many years studying and getting their education. While faith has no place in medicine, trust will always play a role. It is the nature of all human relationships. How does a healthcare provider earn your trust? It should have nothing to do with the number of letters they have after their name, nor the impressiveness of the organizations that they are members of. It should definitely not come from a perceived intellectual superiority.

The following criteria may help you find a medical practitioner with whom you can have a trusting relationship (while it is true that many doctors are female, I have used the male pronoun for simplicity):

- Respect — He respects your opinion and trusts your knowledge of yourself and your body. He also respects your preference for treatment or lack thereof. He understands that the final medical decision is yours and yours alone. He aims for individualized care, with the patient's best interest as the central focus.
- He fully understands and is able to explain the benefits *and risks* of any treatment or diagnostic procedure offered.
- First do no harm — He never offers treatments that are more harmful than the disease. In the case of a mild illness, or especially for prevention, life-threatening treatments will *not* be recommended.
- Doctor's orders — Why are doctors giving orders? Doctors are service providers; they are here to help improve your health. Choose a doctor who advises without expecting blind obedience, not one who commands. Treatment is never given without the patient's consent. He does not employ coercive tactics such as guilt, fear, or intellectual superiority to gain compliance.

- He has thoroughly reviewed and is *actually knowledgeable* about potential side effects of any treatment, and never discounts side effects that the patient experiences. Before proceeding, he questions the efficacy, safety, and necessity of any potentially risky treatment, determining to the greatest degree of certainty whether it will help or harm the patient. Furthermore, he recognizes that side effects are not an acceptable part of treatment, and has enough empathy to realize when his treatments have caused or worsened his patients' suffering and is willing to take responsibility.
- He is open to learning new ideas, and not just from the pharmaceutical complex or the medical authorities and experts, but from everywhere, even and especially his own patients. He is constantly seeking to uncover the truth, and is not simply following the rules blindly. He doesn't rigidly believe in medical rules since he knows that medicine is ever-changing, and what is right today may be wrong tomorrow.
- A lot of doctors say they are too busy and therefore have no time for research. If they are so busy, then they don't need your business. Find a doctor who is less busy and has time to do some independent investigation.

This sort of relationship is never guaranteed with any healthcare provider, but I do believe that good care is impossible without it.

WHO TAKES CREDIT FOR LONGEVITY?

A Myopic View of History

*Up until the twentieth century, few people outlived their thirties; most people lost half their children to childhood diseases; almost nobody experienced heart disease, cancer, or Alzheimer's, but only because almost nobody reached old age. All medicine was quackery: **there was no effective form of medicine in existence to combat illness for over five thousand years.** Then modern medicine entered the scene and saved humanity (cue the celestial music). Thanks to the ingenious scientists of the twentieth century, we now have control over nature (which would otherwise run wild), we have control* *over almost all diseases, and we therefore have longevity...*and I would like to sell you a bridge.

Isn't this what we've all been told? But could there really have been nothing effective to combat disease for most of human history? And are we really to believe that nobody was enlightened enough to understand nature or the human body until the twentieth century? Was the entire history of the world one long dark-age of medical and scientific ignorance, finally culminating in the enlightenment of the modern era? But doesn't every era think that they're the most enlightened in history? Or were the folks of the sixteenth century lamenting their ignorance, just waiting with bated breath for true knowledge of the twentieth century to release them from darkness...?

Considering how fickle modern science is, where each new breakthrough contradicts previously held beliefs, it's hard to imagine that the twentieth and twenty-first centuries are truly the age of undisputed scientific perfection and ultimate truth. Technology is certainly astounding, and new and fascinating discoveries are being made every day. But the ability to observe and understand nature has always existed. Perhaps previous generations had some knowledge of health that is worth preserving. Perhaps they even understood certain aspects of nature *better* that we do. Before modern times and before the creation of modern medicine, were there societies that experienced longevity? Is medical advancement the true key to longevity? Maybe not. What other factors were involved?

When life expectancy is short, some of the following criteria are almost always involved:

- Poverty
- Dire living conditions (such as overcrowding, lack of heat in the winter, and lack of adequate clothing for insulation from the cold)
- Poor hygiene (including unclean living environment, poorly managed sewage, contaminated drinking water, body lice, and rat infestation)
- Malnutrition (such as a diet consisting of only bread — almost completely deficient in all vitamins and minerals) or total famine

- Toxic contamination and pollution especially from industrial waste
- Death due to "childbed fever" in mothers after birth, resulting in many orphaned children who inevitably often died in childhood, resulting in extremely skewed statistics for life expectancy
- Unsafe work conditions
- War

Childbed fever was an infection that occurred in women after giving birth in hospitals. It was the result of infection due to unwashed contaminated hands of doctors, who often attended births straight out of the morgue. Childbed fever was rare for mothers who birthed in their own homes. Wealthy women birthed at home, while impoverished women were forced to birth in dangerous, contaminated hospitals.

In Western society, overcrowding and lack of proper sewage disposal was a direct result of the industrial revolution when society moved en masse into cities seeking their fortune. What they got instead were deplorable living conditions and poverty. Orphaned children were at particular risk of not surviving until adulthood under these conditions.

What I have *not* mentioned as a cause of shortened life expectancy is lack of adequate medicine. Medicine will do next to nothing under the above circumstances. And although there may have been exceptions, most epidemic diseases that decimated societies relied upon the above conditions to spread. In particular, sewage-contaminated drinking water and rat infestation are among the greatest culprits of the spread of disease.

If a goldfish were living in a tank full of filthy sewage, bacteria, and ammonia, would you add antibiotics to the tank? No. If you gave medicine to a fish living in sludge, you would probably hasten its demise. The way to save the fish would be to clean the tank and give it fresh, clean water.

So what is the real reason for longevity today? The same reason for longevity in any generation.

- Prosperity
- Clean living conditions
- Adequate nutrition
- Proper disposal of sewage
- Clean, uncontaminated drinking water
- Minimal pollution
- Adequate clothing
- Sufficient housing
- Protection from harsh weather conditions
- Lack of war and civil unrest

Although modern medicine gives itself a lot of credit for the longevity that society is currently enjoying, it is most probably undeserved. It is and has always been good living conditions that have allowed societies to enjoy longevity. The treatment of disease with medicine is very much after the fact.

EVOLUTION AND GENETICS

In the years I have spent digging through modern medical research, I have come across a fiercely guarded belief in the Theory of Evolution. Despite the many gaps and lack of evidence, evolution is accepted as a scientific certainty. What people do not realize is how much direct influence unproven evolutionary ideology has on medical "progress."

The best example I can think of is genetics. Genetics is, in essence, the "science" of evolution. What geneticists believe is that most diseases are due to arbitrarily occurring genetic defects (called "mutations"), as opposed to preventable environmental factors.

Evolutionists also theorize that these mutations have been responsible for transforming arthropods into thinking human beings. However, geneticists admit that they have yet to come across a single mutation that has *improved* a species. In every case where mutant genes are found, the result is a defect or a disease. So it becomes evident that the theory that genetic mutations could ever have been responsible for advancing a species is a pure leap of faith.

On the other hand, scientists claim that mutations are a necessary part of the evolutionary process, weeding out the genetically unfit. For example, the BRCA gene that supposedly predicts breast cancer risk has been leading many people down a slippery path. Breast cancer has so many clearly evident environmental and lifestyle risk factors that blaming the whole thing on genetics is downright dangerous.

It is dangerous for two reasons:

Firstly, it leads a lot of women to "courageously" pursue life-threatening surgeries. Women are even undergoing sterility-inducing hysterectomies (surgical removal of the uterus) in the prime of their fertile years to prevent a disease they don't even have! (Sterilizing women with a genetic mutation is eerily reminiscent of the eugenics movement of the early twentieth century.) All because of a gene that **may slightly** increase their risk of cancer.[1]

Secondly, cancer can occur almost anywhere in the body, and removing parts may prevent cancer in those areas (because they are no longer there), but it certainly will not prevent cancer elsewhere.

The real way to prevent cancer is to avoid exposure to and consumption of carcinogens, and to build up the immune system so that the body is capable of finding and destroying cancer cells. Genetics completely ignores the environmental causes of disease and renders us powerless victims of fate, at the mercy of state-of-the-art medical advancement.

Geneticists say, "If we can just isolate the gene that causes this problem, then we are only one step away from a cure." Scientists believe that they will soon be able to control the environment through technological advancement. This is not true and will never be true, because as much as they try, science will never overpower nature. Modern medicine's

---

1   H. Gilbert Welch, MD, M.P.H., *Over-Diagnosed*, 2011.

ability to observe phenomena does not usually translate into the ability to control what they are observing.

The media predicts that it is just a matter of time before man develops the technology to cure all disease (and thus live forever?). I am not convinced that nature needs to be fixed, and the idea of man controlling nature should be terrifying to all of us. It seems that modern medicine has it backward: they believe that nature causes disease and that man can cure it through his advancing technological capabilities.

What usually happens is quite the opposite: man causes disease, and only by going back to nature can we reverse the damage. We are living in a highly polluted environment, eating genetically modified or processed junk foods, trans fats, preservatives, artificial colors, flavors, etc. We are exposed to potentially deadly drugs, x-rays, electromagnetism, pesticides, fluoride, heavy metals, and more. All these things cause disease.

I am not trying to scare you; we all do the best we can. I am simply pointing out that before pursuing theoretical genetic factors — and removing parts of your body — why not try to remove disease-causing agents from your surrounding environment? This is actually a lot less frightening.

Our genetics are not set in stone. Rather, the health of our genes and those of our offspring rely heavily on our environment. For example, malnutrition and x-ray exposure are known causes of birth defects. All life forms that produce healthy offspring when properly nourished can produce defective progeny when malnourished or exposed to toxins.[2] Despite the media's strong emphasis on genetics alone as the main cause of disease, there is at best a slight correlation between these ever-changing genetic findings and most diseases.

Now that modern medical intervention is the number-one cause of death in the US, followed by heart disease and cancer,[3] it's time we stopped being intimidated by medical mystique and began taking

---

2   Weston A. Price, DDS, *Nutrition and Physical Degeneration*, 8th edition, Price-Pottenger Nutrition Foundation, 1939–2014.

3   Gary Null, PhD, Carolyn Dean, MD, ND, Martin Feldman, MD, Debora Rasio, MD, and Dorothy Smith, PhD, *Death by Medicine*, 2010.

control of our own health. If we can no longer put our faith in medicine, it's time to look back at the remedies that nature provides, as well as our body's natural healing abilities.

SHOOT FIRST, ASK QUESTIONS LATER

When it comes to preserving one's health, the better we understand our options, the better off we'll be. Whichever path of medicine we choose, barring genuine emergencies, we usually have more time than we are given to get informed. Time is the key — when health problems are presented as urgent and in need of immediate treatment, there's no time to mull things over. On the other hand, when we *can* take the time to figure out the risks and benefits of the treatments being offered, we'll be able to calmly decide which options to pursue. So the first step in becoming an empowered and informed medical consumer is learning to differentiate between genuine medical emergencies, and situations where we have the luxury to make the decision.

Here are some examples of situations that require urgent care, in which there is no time to research:

- Choking or any situation where breathing is compromised
- Anaphylactic reactions
- Acute asthma attack
- Accidents and traumatic injuries
- Poisoning
- Acute stage of heart attack or stroke
- Acute severe bacterial infection that is spreading or in the blood
- Any other life-threatening emergency

Many other conditions are treated as emergencies, but do not in fact require urgent care. Some illnesses *may* be life threatening or may eventually *become* life threatening, but not in a manner of minutes or even days. In these situations, even though we are often told to begin treatment immediately, the truth is that taking a step back and weighing one's options can be more lifesaving than the treatments being offered.

Conditions that should not be treated as medical emergencies:

- Childbirth
- Miscarriage
- Hypertension (chronic)
- Strep throat
- Ear infection
- Chronic asthma
- Cancer diagnosis
- Any other chronic disease

These are just a few examples, but they illustrate the importance of differentiating between genuine emergencies, and situations that may be serious but do not necessitate a blind emergent rush into treatment.

I know that I use cancer as an illustration far too often. But I have a reason: cancer is the most terrifying and disempowering diagnosis a person can receive. Since my goal in writing this book is to inform and empower the medical consumer, I must emphasize a situation where patients are in the greatest need for empowerment. Nevertheless, the following illustration can be applied to many other situations as well.

Every cancer diagnosis is treated as an emergency. Patients are told to begin treatment *immediately*, that even a delay of a few days can be the difference between life and death. Although cancer can be a deadly disease, even the most aggressive and fast-growing cancers do not kill overnight. The rush into treatment can endanger the patient more than the disease itself. Instead of rushing into treatment, take the time to explore the available options. Weigh risks and benefits *before* initiating treatment. Afterward, it's too late. No non-emergent medical decision should be made when one is in a state of fear. When one is uninformed, cancer is much more frightening, and treatment options are severely limited.

Even diagnostic techniques for cancer must be weighed carefully to be certain that they will not cause what they are intended to prevent.

- Mammograms are x-rays, which are a known carcinogen. So mammograms themselves can transform healthy tissue into cancerous tissue. Mammograms also sandwich the breast tissue in a way that may cause a self-contained tumor to burst and metastasize.

- CAT scans are also x-rays, and considering how extensive their coverage is, they expose a lot of the body to x-ray radiation, which, of course, is carcinogenic.
- Biopsy — Most people are unaware of the fact that a biopsy can cause tumors to spread.

> Manipulation of an intact tumor by FNA (fine needle aspiration) or large-gauge needle core biopsy is associated with an increase in the incidence of... metastases, perhaps due in part to the mechanical disruption of the tumor by the needle. The clinical significance of this phenomenon is unclear.[4]

Being knowledgeable is the most important thing you can do for your health — while doctors almost always mean well, the urgency and arbitrarily set time limits for any given treatment often leave patients without the ability to choose. The result of these time constraints and the emergent nature of almost every diagnosis is that patients become vulnerable due to lack of information and lack of time to get informed before treatment is commenced.

The sentiment is that we must act now! But must we? First, we must be sure that the diagnosis is, in fact, correct and that this treatment will be helpful and not harmful. The key is to stop treating every medical diagnosis as an emergency. This is the first step on the path to medical free choice, to avoid becoming a victim of unnecessary treatments and even surgeries — which can have lifelong negative health consequences. Being that the ramifications can be so long lasting, as often as possible we have to take the time to think about our options before jumping into treatment.

4   N.M. Hansen, X. Ye, B.J. Grube, A.E. Giuliano, *Manipulation of the Primary Breast Tumor and the Incidence of Sentinel Node Metastases from Invasive Breast Cancer*, Arch Surg. 2004;139(6):634–640. doi:10.1001/archsurg.139.6.634.

"IS IT REALLY NECESSARY?"

Consider just one example: the cesarean section. Cesareans are so common that the term "unnecesarean" was coined to describe the unprecedented rise in C-sections. (In the US, one in three births is via cesarean, and the US is not breaking any world records. In Brazil, the cesarean rate is over 55 percent! The current trend toward high cesarean rates across the world is unprecedented in history. However, the increase in surgical births has not resulted in better birth outcomes. Countries performing far fewer C-sections are producing healthier infants and mothers.

According to a study in *The Lancet*, "Rate of cesarean delivery was positively associated with postpartum antibiotic treatment and severe maternal morbidity and mortality, even after adjustment for risk factors. Increase in the rate of cesarean delivery was associated with an increase in fetal mortality rates and higher numbers of babies admitted to intensive care for seven days or longer even after adjustment for preterm delivery."

Furthermore, cesarean is major surgery with all the risks involved. One of the reasons I began giving childbirth classes was to put mothers back in control and prevent them from becoming victims of risky medical procedures, unless absolutely necessary. Women who are trying for natural births after cesareans are also most likely to be successful when they are well educated.

Tip: If the doctor says that an emergency C-section is necessary, ask if they can wait an hour or two. If they can, you know it's not a real emergency — take that time to get a second (and third!) opinion. Bringing an experienced doula along can help prevent a lot of unnecessary intervention.

RETAINING CONTROL

In general, when a patient receives a diagnosis and a suggested treatment:

1. Find out more about the diagnosis you've received. It's a good idea to do your *own* research. Read books, find other people who have experience with the treatment being offered to you, especially if it's new. Ask tough questions, and don't proceed until you get satisfactory answers. Find a healthcare provider who understands your concerns and takes you seriously. Don't let anyone convince you that you're not capable of understanding the situation. You are. You have a responsibility to yourself and your family to know all the risks and benefits of *any* medical diagnosis and treatment.

Sometimes, non-diseases are treated as illnesses, turning healthy people into lifelong patients. An important example of this is statin drugs used to lower cholesterol (Lipitor, etc.). Years ago, medical authorities identified an arbitrary cholesterol level as high and as the cause of heart disease. Based on these numbers, they falsely transformed millions of healthy people into cardiac patients. However, in recent history, the public became aware that the cumulative scientific evidence has proven that cholesterol level does not correlate with heart disease.

A 2015 study printed in the British Medical Journal, which analyzed data from studies conducted on 68,094 elderly people, concluded that, "High LDL-C is inversely associated with mortality (i.e., higher "bad" cholesterol is associated with lower death rates) in most people over sixty years. This finding is inconsistent with the cholesterol hypothesis (i.e., that cholesterol, particularly LDL-C, is inherently atherogenic). [In other words, the study finds that cholesterol does not cause fatty deposits in the arteries; that the cholesterol hypothesis is wrong.] Since elderly people with high LDL-C live as long or longer than those with low LDL-C, our analysis provides reason to question the validity of the cholesterol hypothesis."

The researchers recommended reevaluating the use of cholesterol-lowering drugs as a means of heart disease prevention.

Once it was determined that people with high cholesterol are not at greater risk of heart disease, Lipitor should have been removed from the market, since lowering cholesterol does not reduce heart disease risk.

Instead, the drug industry concluded that since cholesterol level does not predict heart disease, the screening process for cardiac patients should be broadened to include other factors (such as weight, blood pressure, and smoking status).

That makes sense. However, with perverted logic, they went on to conclude that people found to be at risk should be prescribed cholesterol medication! So instead of being very bad for business, they manipulated the situation to increase their target market.

To rehash: The "Diet-heart hypothesis" originally postulated that the more cholesterol and saturated fat a person ate, the more atherosclerosis (clogged arteries) they would develop. Thus, foods containing these nutrients (yes, saturated fats and cholesterol are nutrients) were said to cause heart disease. Then, when it was found that dietary intake of saturated fat and cholesterol had no bearing on blood levels of these nutrients, nor any effect on circulation, the "diet" part of the hypothesis was discarded (by those who kept up with the science, anyway).

Still, the belief that cholesterol levels predicted heart disease remained strong, until that too was disproven. Once cholesterol levels were found to be poor predictors of heart disease, and that in fact higher levels of cholesterol seemed to be protective, there could be no justification to view cholesterol levels as a marker for heart disease risk. But if it is not a risk factor for heart disease, then how can cholesterol-lowering medications possibly protect against heart disease?

Once all the pieces of this puzzle have been pieced together, we are left with a rather...puzzling situation.

Whether the diagnosis is strep throat, failure to progress during labor, high cholesterol, or even cancer, whenever possible, take the time to understand the basis of the diagnosis and how it applies to you before proceeding to treatment.

2. Evaluate whether the diagnosis is accurate. Doctors are knowledgeable and well-intentioned but not perfect — and often disagree among themselves. It's okay to question their conclusions. Do you actually have this condition? You may be surprised that if you get a second opinion, you may receive an entirely different diagnosis.

3. Research the treatment you are being offered. What are the risks? Is the treatment more dangerous than the disease? How

common are the side effects? Are the side effects more severe than your current symptoms? Many people get stuck in a vicious cycle where they are taking medications to treat the side effects of their original medications, only to watch their health slowly deteriorate. Often, many of their symptoms are not due to the original disease, but to all the drugs or surgeries they've received to treat it!

4. After weighing the risks of the disease against the risks of the treatment, find out if any effective alternative treatments are available.

In truth, the media rarely gives us a well-rounded picture. Journalists are not particularly well-informed about medical issues and often simply follow the voice of the medical industry, whether right or wrong.

No situation is hopeless, and modern medicine does not hold exclusive rights to healing. *Rather than believing in "cutting-edge" medicine's power to fix theoretical defects in the human body, we'd best start believing in the body's G-d-given ability to heal itself.* Health is not found in the halls of hospitals or in pharmaceutical laboratories. It's in you.

TRUE PREVENTION

A while ago, a friend lent me a book on a specific form of healing. When I returned it to her, I observed that while it was informative, I was disappointed that the author seemed to (almost deliberately) leave out one of the main causative factors for the condition the book was meant to treat. "What does it matter what the cause was?" my friend asked me. "If we have a way to treat the problem, just use the methods regardless of the cause."

There are a few reasons why it is important to understand the true underlying causes of illness. Let's take an example: the "new" problem of peanut allergies, an epidemic that exploded around 1991.

Modern medicine observed the new anaphylactic (deadly allergic) issue and created "awareness." Therefore, they sell EpiPens, create "peanut-free" foods, and educate the public about how to be considerate of all those with peanut allergies. All of this is well-intentioned and sounds quite considerate of those plagued with peanut allergies.

Still, perhaps we should ask the obvious questions: Why are so many children suddenly developing deadly allergies to peanuts, and what can we do to prevent more cases?

One theory, labeled the "Helminth Hypothesis," suggested that it had to do with a *lack* of intestinal worm infestation. This was based on the fact that some isolated primitive groups who happened to have severe worm problems did not experience allergies. Other factors, such as lack of exposure to modern lifestyle and modern medicine were not considered. Interestingly, more recently, parasitic infestation is being blamed for triggering allergies. Which one is it? Perhaps neither.

Other contradictory theories abound, ranging from lack of early exposure to the allergen to excessive early exposure! Most of these theories are equally implausible or contradictory. Why is it so difficult to get to the bottom of this mystery?

Part of the reason appears to be because few researchers are really investing much energy into figuring out *why*. Most of their effort is going toward creating products that will improve the lives of peanut-allergy sufferers — and spreading awareness about the problem. More on this subject later.

Another example is the epidemic of cancer that we are experiencing today. America, with all of its cutting-edge treatments, has one of the highest cancer rates in the world. Modern medicine puts most of its efforts into developing more of what they are already doing (chemotherapy, radiation, and surgery). They also put a lot of effort into "awareness" and early detection. While this is well-intentioned and these treatments can be lifesaving in some cases, nevertheless the current efforts have done little to stem the tide of illness.

THE CANCER INDUSTRY'S BEST-KEPT SECRETS

As the rates of many forms of cancer increase, one may wonder: What is the cause? Some of this increase may be due to the overdiagnosis of cancer, but certainly not all of it. However, the increase in cancer due to overdiagnosis is one of the main reasons that cancer death rates have seemingly gone down in recent years. Because of aggressive screening, people are being diagnosed *earlier*. The result has been a five-year survival rate, which appears as though cancer patients are living longer lives than in previous generations. However, this is not the case; they are simply being *diagnosed* younger, thus living longer with the knowledge that they have cancer.

Since very little has changed over the past century in the mainstream cancer treatments, it's hard to expect any vast improvement in life expectancy for cancer patients. It may come as quite a surprise to many people that chemotherapy, radiation, and surgery have existed for over a century. The changes and improvements have been minor. It's actually rather mysterious why these three treatments have remained modern medicine's *only* defense against cancer when all three are extremely damaging to health and rather unsuccessful in curing cancer. You may have noticed that when using these three treatments, cancer will never be labeled as cured, only in remission.

According to the National Cancer Institute, there has been a significant increase in the overall rate of childhood cancers in recent years — a 27 percent increase since 1975 in kids under age nineteen.[5] Why are more *children* than ever developing cancer today? And my question is: Why aren't they focusing more attention on these important questions? Here's why we should be.

Let's say that Irving's grandmother has multiple sclerosis, and he is her primary caregiver. If Irving finds out that eating yellow jelly beans is the main cause of multiple sclerosis, he will make sure that his grandmother does not eat any more yellow jelly beans. He will also make sure his kids and everyone else in his family stop eating the multiple-sclerosis-causing beans.

Of course, it's never that simple — but the point is that knowing the cause will prevent Irving's grandmother from continuing to poison herself and exacerbate her own condition. It will also prevent others from developing multiple sclerosis from eating yellow jelly beans. Additionally, being aware that yellow jelly beans are the root cause may help heal, since there is a special "yellow jelly bean detoxification program" that is especially powerful for this condition.

---

5   Andy Miller, Brenda Goodman, MA, Hansa D. Bhargava, MD, "Childhood Cancer Rates Are Rising. Why?" WebMD, October 18, 2016.

To summarize, knowing the cause of a disease will:

1. prevent you from reexposing the ill person;
2. prevent other people from being exposed to this potential hazard;
3. often give you the key to true healing.

When we don't understand the underlying mechanisms that have led to a condition, the problem looms much more frightening, intangible and impossible to vanquish. Unmask it, and now we know exactly what we are dealing with. This can open many doors to healing and *true* prevention.

An honest assessment of the true causes of disease takes courage. While we can't always pinpoint the cause of a particular illness, often we can: Many illnesses are largely traceable to tangible causes in our history, lifestyle, diet, etc. Blaming most diseases on genetics (as modern science is apt to do), makes us helpless victims of fate.

DISEASES THAT ARE MORE ENVIRONMENTAL THAN GENETIC

The following is a partial list of diseases that have been labeled by the scientific community as "genetic," when they are in fact largely environmental:

- ADHD
- Asthma
- Allergies
- Cancer
- Autism
- Alzheimer's disease
- Parkinson's disease
- Multiple sclerosis
- Diabetes (certain forms)

The Human Genome Project was a vastly expensive attempt to understand the root source of all disease. It was based on the very shaky presumption that genes are the blueprint of human (and all life-form) development, and that every being's future is already imprinted and predicted in their DNA. The truth is that DNA may be more like a microcosm of the body rather than an oracle; when the body is sick, the DNA is sick. When the body is poisoned (by plastics, lead, mercury, aluminum, drugs, etc.) the DNA is altered. But whether the body expresses healthy or unhealthy traits will depend largely on what is going *into* and going *on in* the body. This is the new field of epigenetics — how genetic expression interplays with the environment.

In truth, we have a lot more control over our health than we realize. As long as we are in the dark about what is making people ill, we are fated to repeat the same mistakes.

Please note that all names and some details in the various accounts presented in this book have been changed to protect the privacy of the individuals.

1

LIVING
SEASONALLY

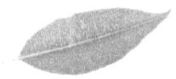

Did you ever wonder why hairy dogs shed in the summer and grow thick coats in the winter? Or why all those skinny mangy cats suddenly look like giant fluff balls during the cold weather? Me neither! It always seemed obvious — G-d, in His infinite kindness, did not want the animals to overheat in the summer or freeze to death in the winter.

When we observe nature, we can learn common sense. If animals were created to sport heavy coats during the winter, maybe there is a reason for it, besides fashion, of course.

SCIENTISTS VS. MOM

Recently, it has been suggested that the parallel between cold weather and frequent infection (colds, flu, etc.) is purely coincidental, going so far as to say that protecting oneself against the elements will not prevent disease. The explanation for why people tend to get sick more during the colder seasons is that people are cooped up together in enclosed spaces for long periods of time (dubbed "the indoor germ theory").

Of course, sometimes disease is transmitted due to poor ventilation and overcrowding, but colds and flu have a lot more to do with the weather, and there is no denying this. People especially tend to get sick when they are not prepared for the weather (i.e., the sunny day forecasted turns into a frigid rainy day — and everyone comes home with a sniffle). People often become ill during season changes — for this very reason. Indeed, the indoor germ theory is slowly losing favor.

Regarding common sense, I believe that mothers have been given a megadose of it. So much so, that even the most prestigious group of scientists cannot stand up to Mother's wisdom. In retrospect, you may recall that your mother *was* always right! If she didn't think that it would be a good idea for Sara to wear her sundress to playgroup on a frigid winter day, even though scientists and Sara may disagree, I put my faith in Mommy.

In addition to the microorganisms involved, exposing one's body to the elements and being unprepared for varying weather conditions can be one of the primary triggers for illnesses like colds and flu. Our body's exterior — our skin layer and our nose and mouth — protect us from contracting illnesses, but they are also the route of entry when we are vulnerable. When we are exposed to cold, windy, or rainy days, our exterior and immune system tries its best to protect us from the elements, but it must work much harder when fighting frigid temperatures.

In recent years, in a (wildly successful) effort to sell (largely ineffective) products such as flu vaccines and antiviral medication, the media has increased the public's fear of disease through campaigns promoting misinformation about the dangers of infectious disease. Sadly, this has done little to stem the tide of illness and promote genuine health.

Most contagious diseases come and go leaving no permanent effect on the body. Besides discomfort or lost time, these diseases pose little risk to people with normal immune function — and taking drugs to "fix" them can sometimes cause more harm than good.

Keep in mind that people get sick most easily when they are worn down. Lack of sleep, an overly sedentary lifestyle, and poor nutrition weaken overall health. A great way to protect yourself during the winter season is by making sure you are not vitamin deficient. Taking supplements such as vitamins C and D$_3$ can boost immune function and prevent negative effects of many contagious diseases.

SUMMER OR WINTER?

While walking through my neighborhood one winter day, I observed some children running jacketless down the street, eating ices. It does not take too much effort to understand why such practices are not healthful.

Where I live, many grocers phase out the frozen snacks by mid-fall, and eventually put the extra freezers into storage for the winter. Recently, however, I have noticed this trend changing. In many super-markets, this seasonal practice is not observed, and ice cream is sold throughout the winter! With the advent of modernity, traditional wisdom and common sense are slipping through our fingers.

Being in sync with the seasons was a part of all traditional cultures. There really was no other choice, since produce varied seasonally. Winter and summer fruits and vegetables were available only during their season. Today, everything is available year-round. This means that we have to take a step back and use our intuition to determine which foods are better for different times of the year.

As a general rule:

- Lightly cooked foods and raw fruits and vegetables are best consumed during the spring and summer. Salad is more appropriate for warmer weather.
- Winter is the best time for warm foods; heavy root vegetables, hearty, thick soups, and larger quantities of chicken and meat. During the winter, avoiding overexposure to the cold includes what we put into our body too. Save ices and cold drinks for the hottest summer days only.

FOOD TEMPERATURE

The importance of temperature is widely unrecognized in modern society, but is central to a healthy diet in traditional medicine. Cold foods, and particularly iced drinks, should be avoided, especially during the winter. The body digests food best when it is warm. Only since the advent of refrigeration have cold and frozen foods become so readily available.

Digestive enzymes only function at body temperature, so by consuming cold, and especially frozen, foods, your digestive system will inevitably have the job of warming up the food so that it can be processed. For some people (particularly those with cold or weaker constitutions) warming cold food to body temperature can be very draining or near impossible, in which case the food may just end up passing through undigested.

> Miriam came to me with her infant, who was experiencing terrible diaper rash. Miriam reported that the baby was on formula, and that she used water from the water cooler to make his bottles. I told her that the same way that mother's milk is warm, bottle-fed babies require their food warmed as well. Giving an infant cold food can be particularly damaging to an already delicate digestive system.

While the thought of drinking room temperature beverages may be unappetizing to some people, it is actually quite easy to get accustomed to, as it is what the body naturally needs. Many people report that once they accustom themselves to room temperature beverages, iced drinks lose their appeal (with the possible exception of the hottest summer days).

FOOD PREPARATION

There is a certain school of thought in the West that believes that a diet consisting of primarily raw foods is ideal. The understanding is that the cooking process removes some of the nutrients found in raw foods.

It all depends. A raw diet can be cleansing for overweight individuals and those with a strong digestive system. However, it is not recommended for those with weak digestion. To put it simply, we are not cows, and our lack of four stomachs makes it difficult to process very large quantities of uncooked fibrous foods.

The right diet can be very individual; it varies greatly from one person to the next. As a general rule, most people can digest raw food within reason (especially during the summer), but many people need cooked food to make digestion and absorption easier. Although the cooking process may reduce nutritional content to some extent, it will make the nutrients more digestible, which means that you will get more out of the food once it is even lightly cooked. Quick-steaming is a great way to prepare vegetables. Steaming will make them more digestible while still retaining the bulk of their nutrients.

Some people also do really well juicing fresh fruits and vegetables. Juicing breaks the food down into small enough parts to ease digestion. Most of us can judge healthful food choices and the ideal way to prepare foods by paying attention to how our bodies respond to the different things we eat. A food that gives energy to one person may make another person feel weak and tired. No food is good for everyone, and different diets work for different people. Often, if we pay attention to our body's responses, we can figure out which food choices are health promoting for us.

Here are some symptoms to look for after eating, to help you judge whether a food is bad for you:

- Bad taste in your mouth, or bad breath
- Feeling lethargic and tired
- Feeling gassy or bloated
- Diarrhea
- Constipation (though this is not immediate and it may be difficult to pinpoint a specific food)
- Heartburn and indigestion
- Stomach pain
- Phlegm in the back of the throat

Diet may not be the only cause of the above symptoms. However, in cases where certain foods trigger one or more of the above symptoms, removing those foods will be essential to improving health. It may even be all that is needed.

Meir read about a healing diet that suggested eating twelve servings of raw fruits and vegetables each day.

> *It sounded good to him, so he started the diet. Guess what? His entire digestive system quit. He came to me with what appeared on the surface as constipation. I would call it exhaustion — Meir has a weaker digestive system (not a stomach of steel). He did well on cooked or warmed food. This diet was totally inappropriate for his constitution, and it took him a few weeks to recover normal digestive function.*

The above story is demonstrative of the problem with raw-food diets, or any other single-minded dietary solution. They do not take into account individual differences and the fact that a diet that can be great for one person may be terrible for somebody else.

2

SUNBURN

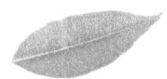

A few years ago, I was discussing with a neighbor my concerns about carcinogenic ingredients in sunscreen. She quickly responded, "I would not play around. My kids recently got terrible sunburns after only a few minutes in the summer sun!"

The currently accepted understanding is that ultraviolet (UV) light reaches us in two main forms, UVA and UVB:

- UVA is harmful radiation; it penetrates more deeply into the skin and can cause cellular damage.
- UVB is what helps your body synthesize vitamin D.

There are several problems with sunscreen.

1. In addition to blocking harmful UVA radiation, sunscreen also blocks health-promoting UVB rays.
2. Most sunscreens contain known carcinogens like oxybenzone or octyl methoxycinnamate,[6] which can also cause cellular damage.

---

6   Ty Bollinger, *Cancer — Step Outside the Box*, 5th edition, 2011.

Ironically, these products tend to deteriorate and become *more* carcinogenic when exposed to sunlight. The chemical ingredients in sunscreen are readily absorbed through the skin.

We are left in a quandary. On the one hand, sunlight has the potential to cause severe sunburns and cellular damage. On the other hand, most sunscreens contain carcinogenic ingredients.

This leads us to a few questions:

1. Is sun exposure good or bad for our health?
2. Is there a reason why some people burn more easily (like my neighbor's kids) while others are not affected negatively by sun exposure?
3. Is there anything we can do to safely prevent sun damage without using toxic sunscreens?

SUN EXPOSURE PREVENTS CANCER

Incredibly, populations in areas that are exposed to more sunlight have lower cancer rates than areas with low sun exposure. So, contrary to popular belief, sunlight is more likely to *prevent* cancer than *cause* it!

The main reason for the inverse relationship between sunlight and cancer is probably that the sun helps the skin produce vitamin D, which plays a role in regulating cholesterol synthesis and calcium absorption, among other things. Even if one consumes enough calcium, if vitamins D and K_2 are inadequate, most of the calcium will not be absorbed and distributed properly. Calcium is essential for normal cell function. Calcium deficiency can result in a malfunction in DNA syntheses, a key first step in the production of cancer cells.[7]

In the middle of the day, the ratio of UVB (the good rays) to UVA (the bad ones) is highest. A daily dose of fifteen to thirty minutes of sun exposure is probably sufficient for vitamin D synthesis. The one caveat is to avoid sunburn. Sunburns are the real risk of sun exposure, and the means by which the sun can promote cellular damage.

---

7   Robert R. Barefoot, Carl J. Reich, MD, *The Calcium Factor*, 5th edition, 2002.

During the winter months (and for those living in less sunny northern climates), insufficient sunlight is a real health risk. This is why many people take supplements when their sun exposure is insufficient. Which to use?

- Cod liver oil is the best choice.
- A good second choice is an oil-based D^3 supplement.
- Milk and many vitamin supplements contain synthetic D^2, which is worthless.

WHAT ABOUT SUNBURN?

Despite the sun's ability to prevent cancer, the threat of UVA rays causing sunburn and cellular damage is still real. So how do we maximize the health benefits of sunlight while minimizing the risk of burns?

Natural Sunscreens

It should come as no surprise that nature has produced effective sunscreens that are far safer than most commercially available options:

Aloe Vera is a plant that grows ubiquitously in Israel, but is available throughout the world. The fresh squeezed gel can be applied before sun exposure, and is even effective in treating all kinds of burns.

Another excellent option is pure **coconut oil**. For generations, the Melanesian natives of the hot tropical South Sea Islands used coconut oil for sun and rain protection. Because it is waterproof, the oil can also be used when swimming.[8]

Why do some people burn while others don't?

Aside from skin tone, there are certain nutritional factors that can reduce our risk of sunburn. Luckily, we can increase our sun tolerance using some of the following:

Vitamin D: Adequate dosage of vitamin D can prevent sun damage. So, remarkably, regular, moderate sun exposure can actually prevent sunburn! Taking cod liver oil or an oil-based D_3 supplement throughout

---

8   Weston A. Price, DDS, *Nutrition and Physical Degeneration*, 8th edition, Price-Pottenger Nutrition Foundation, 1939–2014.

the winter will ensure adequate levels. The USDA's recommended 600 IU of D_3 is far from sufficient. Many third-party researchers have found that at least 2,000–6,000 IU of D_3 are needed to prevent disease.

Tomatoes: Lycopene, found mostly in cooked tomatoes, has been shown to reduce the risk of sun damage. A positive effect was found in women who consumed 55 grams of tomato paste daily, which is just over three tablespoons.

Saturated fat: Increase your intake of saturated fats (found in butter, palm oil, coconut oil, and animal products) and reduce polyunsaturated fats (PUFA) such as canola and other vegetable oils. Though popular belief is that saturated fats are bad for you and PUFAs are good, mounting evidence suggests that just the opposite is true. Unlike PUFAs, saturated fats are more stable and do not degrade when exposed to high heat. Mouse studies have shown that increased intake of saturated fat will decrease melanoma growth.

Green tea: A well-known health food, green tea has been shown to inhibit skin tumor development and prevent DNA damage. Applying green tea extracts directly to the skin can also provide sun protection.[9]

Proanthocyanidins: Found in wine, grape seeds, blueberries, hazelnuts, pistachios, and barley, these have been effective in preventing UV damage in hairless rodents. A recent study found that people who supplemented with grapeseed extract (high in anthocyanidins) had a significantly lower risk of skin cancer.[10]

The risks of sunlight come from sunburn — this is where cellular damage can occur. If you spend lots of time indoors and don't get much sun, take some of the precautions listed above before sun exposure. Don't be afraid of the sun; just be wise about getting sunlight while avoiding sunburn. Lack of sunlight causes far more disease than too much sun.

In summary:

- We need sunlight, particularly UVB rays. Lack of sun exposure can make us sick, both physically and mentally.

---

9   Mark Sisson, *8 Natural Ways to Prevent a Sunburn (And Sunscreen's Not One of Them)*, 2011.
10   Ibid.

- Most sunscreens contain numerous carcinogenic chemicals, so choose ones with only natural ingredients. Some researchers believe that sunscreen causes more cancer than the sun.
- It is especially important to avoid sunburns; that's where the dangers of sun exposure lie.

One final note: One of the greatest dangers of summer can be dehydration and heatstroke. So while you enjoy the great outdoors, don't forget to keep properly hydrated. Also, if you will be out in the sun for an extended period of time, wear a light-colored cotton hat to protect from heatstroke.

3

BREAKFAST

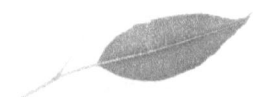

I was asked by a magazine to write an article about breakfast being the most important meal of the day. Being someone who does not like to espouse the opinions of others as my own, especially in the absence of compelling justification *for* those opinions, I made it the goal of my research for the article to answer the question: "Is breakfast *truly* the most important meal of the day?"

The same question can be asked about salt: Is salt really bad for you? (Since I have not covered this topic in this book, I will tell you in short: no. But refined table salt is. Unrefined salts with minerals intact actually contain calcium, magnesium, potassium, and more, which are, in fact, very good for the heart.) There are many widely held beliefs that we take for granted to be based on reality. However, when we delve beneath the surface we find that many of these beliefs have been carried by inertia (or some other force), but not truth. I have made it my job to differentiate fact from myth. Back to breakfast:

We have been told that:

> Breakfast kick-starts your metabolism, helping you burn calories throughout the day. It also gives you the energy you need to get things done, and helps you focus at work or at school. Those are just a few reasons why it's the most important meal of the day. Many studies have linked eating breakfast to good health, including better memory and concentration...[11]

According to the federal government's US Dietary Guidelines, eating breakfast is recommended every day because "not eating breakfast has been associated with excess body weight."[12] Is this doctrine based on verifiable evidence? Recently, many scientists have scrutinized the current belief that eating breakfast has a positive effect on weight control. There are strong doubts whether there is adequate evidence to make this claim.

THE MAIN MEAL AROUND THE WORLD

Traditionally, different cultures have emphasized different meals as their main one. In many European nations and in Israel, lunch is the main meal today, while dinner and breakfast are on the sidelines. In the US, where the media has been espousing breakfast as the most important meal for decades, the main meal is, of course...dinner! A glimpse at history reveals that many societies *ate only two meals a day*. Some even ate only one!

According to food historian Caroline Yeldham,

> **Breakfast as we know it didn't exist for large parts of history**. The Romans didn't really eat it, usually consuming only one meal a day around noon. In fact, breakfast was actively frowned upon.

---

11 "Breakfast: Is It the Most Important Meal?" Reviewed by Kathleen M. Zelman, MPH, RD, LD, WebMD, February 23, 2016.
12 Peter Whoriskey, "The science of skipping breakfast: How government nutritionists may have gotten it wrong," *Washington Post*, August 10, 2015.

> The Romans believed it was healthier to eat only one meal a day...They were obsessed with digestion, and eating more than one meal was considered a form of gluttony. This thinking impacted on the way people ate for a very long time.
>
> The ancient Greeks [known for their physical and mental prowess] ate but two meals a day. The same was true of the ancient Hebrews and it is the custom of some of the best fighting races in India today.[13]

Now, let's consider how life according to the Torah affects our eating habits. Firstly — at least for men, who are obligated in time-bound mitzvos (commandments) — prayer comes first. So even if you'll be eating breakfast, it won't be first thing in the morning. If you look at the festivals, things get even stranger. On Shabbos (Sabbath) day, there is lunch and *shalosh seudos* (the third meal; the first is Friday night). So on the holiest day of the week, the day that gives us a glimpse into the World to Come, we are utterly skipping the most important meal of the day?

Will any breakfast do?

While breakfast campaigns have been successful in guilting many people into eating *something*, there are very few (non-retired) persons who sit down for a full-blown feast first thing in the morning.

So realistically speaking, is that granola bar that you ate "hands free" as you sped to work, or the iced coffee you nearly spilled in your lap really doing something important for your health? What about children's breakfast? Is it essential for their health to consume that bowl of multicolored sugar loops floating in skim milk?

THE SCIENCE

Combing through the available research, you will find that claims about the supreme importance of breakfast, specifically that eating

---

13   Mike O'Donnell, "Old Wisdom on Daily Meal Frequency, Why Are You Eating So Much?" theiflife.com.

breakfast helps with weight control, are based on observational (aka "weak") studies. The belief in breakfast was based on the fact that overweight people tend to skip breakfast. What is missing is the evidence proving a direct cause-and-effect relationship. The fact that there is a tendency for obese individuals to skip breakfast does not prove that skipping breakfast causes obesity. Recently, various researchers decided to test the breakfast hypothesis using higher quality study designs.

One randomized controlled trial was conducted on 309 participants who were overweight and obese, but otherwise healthy. Two groups were randomly assigned to eat or skip breakfast over a period of four months, with the only criteria measured being weight loss. The results were surprising. In the words of the researchers, "Contrary to widely espoused views, this had no discernible effect on weight loss in free-living adults who were attempting to lose weight." After reviewing the existing evidence on the subject, the researchers added, "The effectiveness of adopting these recommendations for reducing body weight is unknown."[14]

RIGID BUT BASELESS DIETARY GUIDELINES

Every five years, the US Dietary Guidelines are updated by its advisory committee. What may come as a surprise, calling the credibility of nutritional doctrine into question, was the recent retraction of many fiercely guarded nutritional beliefs. As of 2015, the advisory committee called for dropping the long-standing warning about dietary cholesterol, which had long plagued the egg industry,[15] as recent evidence unequivocally demonstrates that blood cholesterol levels are not correlated with dietary intake of cholesterol.[16]

Additionally, prominent studies have recently contradicted the government warnings about the dangers of salt. Also, according to critics, the government's long-standing condemnation of foods rich in

---

14   E. J. Dhurandhar et al., "The effectiveness of breakfast recommendations on weight loss: a randomized controlled trial," *The American Journal of Clinical Nutrition*, 2014.

15   Peter Whoriskey, *Washington Post*, 2015.

16   Kendrick, Malcolm, MD, *The Great Cholesterol Con*, 2007.

saturated fats was based on weak science.[17] Saturated fats have been baselessly lumped together with trans (partially hydrogenated) fats, when, in reality, the two have vastly different molecular properties and effects on the body.[18]

Regarding breakfast, the 2010 Dietary Guidelines committee announced: "Modest evidence suggests that children who do not eat breakfast are at increased risk of overweight and obesity...The evidence is stronger for adolescents." As for adults, the evidence was described as "inconsistent."[19]

This weak endorsement was enough to get the federal agencies who write the guidelines (the US Department of Agriculture and the Department of Health and Human Services) to continue pushing the breakfast agenda with vigor. The recommendation to eat breakfast as a means to protect against obesity became part of the 2010 Dietary Guidelines.

Linda Van Horn, a professor of nutrition and preventive medicine at Northwestern University, was chair of the 2010 advisory committee. She explained that the amount of evidence available at the time was "limited," and noted that "regardless of the evidence, though, it might be important for you to recognize the value of eating breakfast due to its frequent inclusion of higher fiber containing foods." In fact, fiber is an ingredient that is lacking in the diet of many Americans. Nevertheless, in 2015, the committee made no updates to their breakfast guidelines. The research is still lacking but the advice remains steadfast that breakfast has some supreme importance. But how can we be sure of this when the scientific evidence remains so shaky?

David Allison of the University of Alabama-Birmingham has recently become one of the foremost critics of what he believes is the misuse of nutritional research. He recently compiled a list of five randomized controlled trials that investigated links between breakfast and obesity. Among these five studies, he found that none offered clear evidence

---

17   Peter Whoriskey.
18   Enig, Mary G. PhD, *Know Your Fats*, 2000.
19   Peter Whoriskey.

that skipping breakfast leads to weight gain. Mostly, it seemed, skipping breakfast made no difference.[20]

This is a far cry from breakfast being the most important meal of the day. So it appears that the evidence for breakfast as a means to prevent obesity is very weak. It is balanced by better-designed studies that show that whether one eats breakfast or not has no real effect on weight control. In terms of the other health benefits, science does not clearly differentiate whether healthy people (or health-conscious people) tend to eat breakfast or if the breakfast itself is what makes them healthy. So we still do not know whether eating breakfast actually influences health.

It does seem that breakfast is a very individual choice. Some people report that if they do not eat first thing in the morning, it literally ruins their whole day.

> *Whenever I don't eat breakfast early enough, I feel like my whole day is thrown off. I'm grouchy, lethargic, and nauseous until I do eat. I lose the whole morning, and much of the afternoon as well, even after I've eaten. And I'm hungry the rest of the day, no matter how much I eat for lunch. I think I actually end up consuming more calories in a day than if I would have eaten breakfast.*
>
> —Rachel G., a young mother

Others have told me that they have no appetite in the morning and cannot force themselves to eat. One woman told me that she starts her day with a tea. She eats brunch a few hours later. So it seems like there can be no hard-and-fast rule that applies to everyone.

INTERMITTENT FASTING?

An article on breakfast would not be complete without mentioning the recent trend of intentionally skipping or delaying breakfast, known as "intermittent fasting." Just to mention the obvious, the name of the

---

20   Ibid.

morning meal is "break-fast," implying that we have been fasting up until this point.

The reasoning behind intermittent fasting is that without actually reducing overall calorie consumption, by eating during a smaller window of time, you can encourage weight loss. Weight loss is achieved with intermittent fasting because the body will only start burning off stored fat once digestion is complete. So by stretching the interval between dinner and breakfast, you can lose weight without restricting food intake (just timing), although, in reality, fasting will ultimately lead to reduced calorie consumption, simply because people who practice intermittent fasting get used to eating less often. When they do eat, they do not make up for lost time, but rather consume normal quantities. In fact, most people who practice intermittent fasting find that their appetites are greatly reduced, they are hungry less often, and experience satiety sooner. There is still much debate about the benefits of delaying your first meal and exactly how long to wait before eating.[21]

You can experiment with the following guidelines to help test this method for yourself. Firstly, more important than skipping breakfast is not eating after dinner, a meal that should preferably take place a good few hours before bedtime. Not eating after dinner should give you at least a twelve-hour break from food. This is the starting point. You can increase the space between dinner and breakfast to thirteen or fourteen hours, if that is workable for you.[22] Should hunger arise after dinner, you can munch on fresh vegetables or have an unsweetened beverage.

> *I tried intermittent fasting and noticed that after a few days of delaying breakfast, my energy levels improved! I now eat two large filling meals during the day, which makes my life easier, as I have fewer meals to plan and prepare. I am not eating less, just less often.*
>
> —Mark S., *a long-time dieter*

---

21   Jensen, Pernille, naturopath, "Why It's Okay to Skip Breakfast," *Huffington Post*, 2015.
22   Ibid.

I contacted Dr. David Ludwig, MD, PhD, nutritional researcher at Harvard Medical School and author of the weight-loss book *Always Hungry?* to ask him what he knows about intermittent fasting.

Dr. Ludwig: The evidence basis to support intermittent fasting is very *limited*, with virtually no long-term trials. And people differ greatly in their ability to tolerate fasting, so it's critical to pay attention to your body's responses. For those who can tolerate it, intermittent fasting may provide significant metabolic benefits, such as improved insulin sensitivity. In addition, fasting results in the production of ketones, considered by some a sort of super fuel for brain and body.

YT: So all those warnings about the dangers of ketone bodies (and low- or no-carb diets) are baseless?

Dr. L: Ketones are normal and natural, either when fasting or eating little carbohydrate. Both have been with us for [a] long [time].

YT: Do you recommend intermittent fasting for weight loss?

Dr. L: Intermittent fasting...won't work for everyone. Ultimately, many of the benefits of fasting can be obtained simply by reducing intake of total carbohydrate and/or fast-digesting carbohydrates — including processed grains, potato products, and added sugars.

> *Now that I understand how intermittent fasting works by using your body's fat stores for energy only when your stomach is empty, I understand why my worst (Jewish) fast days were the ones when I awoke before dawn to eat something. Instead of my body making use of stored energy during the fast, by eating an early breakfast I had just alerted my metabolism to expect more food soon. So I was starving all day on those fasts!*
>
> —Meir S., a young father

Having a drink can be an excellent way to start your day. Tea, water with fresh lemon, or even coffee (preferably without sugar) may be taken if you don't experience an energy crash from caffeine. Then, wait until you have an appetite before you eat. Try to eat sitting down (preferably at a table) rather than on the run. Eating during stressful activity may lead to insulin resistance, weight gain, indigestion, and other health problems.

In light of the scarcity of evidence proving the sanctity of breakfast, there is no need to force yourself to eat before you feel hungry. Consider irritability, weakness, or lethargy as signs that you are hungry ("hangry").[23] This mood change is a message that your blood sugar is low and that your body needs food as soon as possible. If this is your tendency, try to eat before your mood sours.

WHAT BREAKFAST?

Finally, let's talk about the content of your breakfast. If breakfast consists of any form of "frosted" or neon cereal, mislabeled as food, there is serious doubt regarding the "importance" of this meal. It would probably be better to skip breakfast than eat colorful sugar first thing in the morning. Avoid foods with added sugar, like super-sweet low-fat yogurts, sugary granola bars, oatmeal packets, and cold cereal.

Reduced-fat foods are often very high in sugar to balance out the lousy taste. These foods will destabilize your blood sugar, cause constant hunger and cravings, and lead to the prediabetic condition known as insulin resistance.[24] To balance your blood sugar, traditional wisdom (backed by recent evidence) tells us to take the sugar and refined carbs out and put the saturated fats (like butter and coconut oil) back in.[25]

If breakfast has any special importance, it probably comes from the fact that it is undiluted by anything else in your digestive tract. So unhealthy choices may have a particularly strong effect, as the chemicals or sugars will be quickly absorbed, given your empty stomach. Therefore, it is advisable to stay away from artificial flavors, sweeteners, colors and preservatives, and stick with unrefined, wholesome, real foods.

Eat fresh vegetables, nuts, and seeds. Many people tolerate fresh fruit as well. Eat salad with a generous amount of wholesome dressing (such as one based on olive oil and fresh lemon juice, or *techinah*). Avocadoes are packed with nutrients and are extremely satiating. Don't

---

23   Ibid.
24   David Ludwig, MD, PhD, *Always Hungry?* 2016.
25   Mary G. Enig, PhD, S.Fallon, *Eat Fat, Lose Fat*, 2004.

cheat yourself and eat only half an avocado because you feel guilty about the fat. On a diet low in refined carbs and sugar, avocado will give you sustained energy and satiety; it won't make you fat.[26] [27]

Eggs are an excellent choice for a quick and filling meal, even for people diagnosed with high cholesterol.[28] It is now well understood that foods with cholesterol do not damage the arteries.[29] [30] Many people report that after eating meals with adequate fat (as opposed to sugary "fast" carbs), they experience long-lasting energy and satiety, and fewer sweet cravings. The need for sweet comes from the blood-sugar dropping rapidly. This can be stabilized with good fats and other unrefined whole foods.

If you tolerate dairy, it is even okay to eat butter, cheese, and full-fat dairy products that lead to long-lasting satiety due to their blood-sugar stabilizing effects.[31] [32] Instead of putting skim milk and sugar in your coffee, try whole milk or cream and no sugar; you may be pleasantly surprised, firstly by the good taste and later by the longer-lasting energy boost you will get from an unsweetened whole-milk beverage. Many low-sugar diets recommend snacking on bittersweet chocolate with 70 percent cocoa, which can be very satisfying.

If you have a strong need for grains, choose rolled or steel cut oats; instead of sweetening them, try making them savory with salt and butter. Or choose another "slow" (digesting) carbohydrate, such as whole-grain or sourdough bread. You can also eat legumes, such as beans, nuts, seeds, and chickpeas. These are great combined with salads and olive oil.

If you are buying breakfast on the go, consider purchasing a cleansing and nutritious vegetable juice or a fruit/vegetable smoothie, with a nut or seed butter (such as almond or sesame) or another natural fat, like

26   Ludwig.
27   Enig.
28   Ibid.
29   Kendrick.
30   Uffe Ravnskov, MD, PhD, *The Cholesterol Myths*.
31   Ludwig.
32   Enig.

dairy cream, avocado, or unrefined oil. Or you can try an unsweetened whole-fat yogurt or *leben*. You can throw in some fresh fruit for sweetness, and nuts or seeds for long-lasting satiety. In a bind, you can try 100 percent fruit preserves for your yogurt. This may not be much better than sugar, but it's a start.

Save cold breakfast cereals for emergencies only, and give kids whole milk rather than skim. Even unsweetened boxed cereals are the farthest thing from staff of life. They are processed using machinery with high heat and chemicals, which can denature (spoil) the grains and strip the product of its vital nutrients. These nutrients are then replaced with artificial substitutes, which may not be absorbed well by the body. The less processed and the closer it is to homemade, the better.

Breakfast habits vary from culture to culture and from one individual to the next. It seems that you can do whatever works best for you and your family and gives you the most long-lasting energy. Breakfast is certainly not the most important meal of the day for everyone, but it may be for you. You know yourself. Follow your body's cues, and you will find your answer.

4

FAT

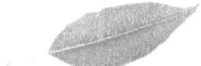

During the past fifty years, fat content in foods has been blamed for making people fat. Since fat has more calories per gram (fat has nine calories versus carbohydrates and protein, which have four), nutritionists and doctors advise restricting fat to stave off obesity. To that end, an entire industry has developed devoted to removing naturally occurring fats from foods and marketing them as "low fat" and therefore dietetic.

As more and more people (including many dieticians) are realizing, this is a mistaken and scientifically invalidated hypothesis.

The undeserved ban of healthy fats has made weight loss difficult, if not impossible for many people, and the fear of fats may be a major contributor to the epidemic of anorexia today. People who cut fat out of their diets often find that they are starving, and their diets are nearly impossible to maintain. Fat-free diets starve the body, and your body will tell you, "I am malnourished! Feed me the foods I need!" As we train our minds to ignore our body's hunger messages (for fat) and, despite this, *still* do not lose weight, some end up abstaining from nearly all food as the only viable weight-loss plan!

Healthy fats are **not** the cause of obesity or heart disease.

Which are the healthy fats? Sometimes, they are the ones we have been told are unhealthy! That is, up until recently, when trans fats finally received the notoriety they deserve. Mary Enig was one of the pioneering researchers who nearly single-handedly proved that trans fats (like margarine and shortening) were the real source of illness, while naturally occurring saturated fats were safe and nutritionally vital. Her revealing research is the reason why many US states have banned hydrogenated/trans fats in manufactured foods.[33]

WHERE'S THE UNADULTERATED COCOA?

I recently noticed that the supermarket shelves were bursting with packages of low-fat cocoa powder. I scoured the baking section to find some unadulterated cocoa and thankfully found one package buried all the way in the back of the shelf. Out of sheer curiosity, I took the two packages and held them side by side to compare their calorie count. I was shocked and temporarily stumped to see that the low-fat cocoa had almost the same number of calories per one hundred-gram serving as the full-fat cocoa.

Looking closer at the label, I realized that while the fat had been reduced, the carbohydrate count had increased, rendering the calorie reduction negligible. Suffice it to say, I bought the full-fat cocoa (even though I didn't need it) out of fear that the low-fat product would soon push its unaltered counterpart off the supermarket shelves.

This is just one example of how the low-fat craze is making people eat less healthy food — and isn't helping them lose the weight.

DAIRY AND MOTHER'S MILK

When dairy products are skimmed of their fat to create "dietetic" products, the milk fat is then used to make valuable products like butter and cream. The unpalatable watery substance that remains is usually thickened with milk protein or other thickeners so that it resembles the texture of whole milk, as opposed to white water. The false notion that saturated fat and cholesterol are unhealthy has even led many parents

---

33   Mary G. Enig, *Know Your Fats: The Complete Primer for Understanding the Nutrition*, 2000.

to feed their youngsters dairy products whose fat has been partially or completely removed.

The practice of giving children a low-fat diet can be dangerous, as brain and body development rely on fat and cholesterol (the same is true in the elderly, who need cholesterol for proper brain function). Consider the fat and cholesterol content in mother's milk (average): Total fat: 4.4%, Saturated fat: 2%, Cholesterol: 14mg. This is higher than "whole" cow's milk. In fact, goat's milk, which is considered nutritionally superior to cow's milk, has a similar fat content to mother's milk. If mother's milk provides 4.4%, how could we expect our children to receive balanced nourishment from 1% skim milk?

APPLESAUCE CAKE?

About twenty years ago, it was all the rage to replace oil with applesauce in pastries. This created a product that was very high in carbohydrates and nearly fat-free. When you take the fat out of a cake and put in applesauce, you have just created a high-carb — and fast-carb — food. This pastry will give you a quick sugar high, followed by an energetic crash, as the "fast carbs" will be out of your bloodstream quickly. Believe it or not, if that cake had contained fat (especially saturated fat like butter or coconut oil), the fat content would have helped stabilize the blood sugar, possibly for hours afterward. By vilifying butter and then, later on, all fats, we have created a recipe for disaster (pun intended). Once again, the low-fat craze makes us unhealthier, hungrier, and — ultimately — fatter.

EAT THE FAT, LOSE THE CAKE

Imagine the sacrifice we have been making eating such dreadful foods in the name of weight loss! If you lose weight by eating fat-free, "fast carb" applesauce cake, you are the exception. Ironically, if you really want to lose weight, throw out the cake and the applesauce, but keep the butter! Stabilizing your blood sugar with saturated fats will keep you satiated and prevent sugar cravings. When it comes to weight loss, it is the sugar and the fast carbs that are the biggest problem, not fat.

BUTTER AND WEIGHT LOSS

When you eat dairy, whole-fat products are better for you. Whole-fat dairy is simply healthier and more balanced than low-fat or skimmed milk products. Just compare dairy to other foods, such as whole grains and unpeeled fruits and vegetables, and it becomes apparent that whole, unadulterated foods are usually nutritionally superior to their processed counterparts.

As we will see, recent evidence shows that whole-fat dairy products are not only better for you; they can actually help you lose weight. For once, you will be able to make your diet more healthful and better tasting simultaneously!

THE EVIDENCE IS CLEAR

Numerous studies have found that not only is low-fat dairy not good for you, but eating it actually causes weight gain. Swedish researchers found that middle-aged men who consumed high-fat milk, butter, and cream were significantly less likely to become obese over a twelve-year period of time, compared with men who never or rarely ate high fat dairy.[34]

In a meta-analysis of sixteen studies, published in the *European Journal of Nutrition*, researchers found that, "Evidence does not support the hypothesis that high-fat dairy foods contribute to obesity and heart disease risk. In most of the studies, high-fat dairy was associated with a lower risk of obesity."[35]

Another study of children, published in the *British Medical Journal*'s Archive of Diseases in Childhood, found that a diet containing low-fat milk was associated with *more* weight gain (a higher body mass index — BMI) over time. "One-percent [or] skim-milk drinkers had higher BMI z-scores than 2 percent [or] whole-milk drinkers. In multivariable analyses, increasing fat content in the

---

34 S. Holmberg, A. Thelin, "High dairy fat intake related to less central obesity: a male cohort study with 12 years' follow-up," *Scand J Prim Healthcare*. 2013 Jun;31(2):89-94. doi: 10.3109/02813432.2012.757070. Epub 2013 Jan 15. ncbi.nlm.nih.gov/pubmed.

35 M. Kratz, T. Baars, S. Guyenet, "The relationship between high-fat dairy consumption and obesity, cardiovascular, and metabolic disease," *Eur J Nutr*, 2013 Feb;52(1):1–24. doi: 10.1007/s00394-012-0418-1. Epub 2012 Jul 19. ncbi.nlm.nih.gov.

type of milk consumed was inversely associated with BMI z-score." Meaning, higher fat milk was associated with lower weight!

They concluded: "Consumption of 1 percent [or] skim milk is more common among overweight/obese preschoolers, potentially reflecting the choice of parents to give overweight/obese children low-fat milk to drink. Nevertheless, 1 percent [or] skim milk does not appear to restrain body weight gain between two and four years of age..."[36]

According to the authors, the results of these studies were a real surprise to them; they had been expecting the opposite outcome.

How does drinking skim milk make kids fatter?

A diet lacking in saturated fats will cause sugar and carbohydrate cravings and a lack of satiety, which will usually result in overeating. Grains and sugar are what make most people fat. Include more butter and whole-milk products in your diet and your sugar cravings will diminish.

Olympic athletes in ancient Greece would drink a bowl full of cream before a competition to give them strength and endurance. Cream was used in this manner because it stabilizes blood sugar for an extended period of time. A diet that is high in saturated fat will prevent ups and downs in insulin. A low-fat diet can cause blood-sugar imbalances and contribute to diabetes and hypoglycemia. So if you include foods with saturated fat, such as butter, in your diet, this will stabilize your blood-sugar and insulin levels and promote long-lasting satiety and help you lose weight!

TRANS FATS

In the 1920s, a new food was introduced, which was free of choles-terol and saturated fat. Touted as a health food, modern society was duped into wholeheartedly embracing "hydrogenated fats," such as margarine and shortening. Now known as trans fats, these supposed health foods have recently been unmasked for their noxious properties, even being banned from the prepared-food market in some US states.

---

36 R.J. Scharf, R.T. Demmer, DeBoer MD, "Longitudinal evaluation of milk type consumed and weight status in preschoolers," *Archives of Disease in Childhood* 2013;98:335–340.

These "factory fats" have been a huge contributor to obesity, cancer, and many other diseases. The immediate lesson: avoid trans fats (hydrogenated fats). The larger lesson: Don't immediately trust new and artificial solutions — give them a chance to be tested over time, which will often show that they do more harm than good.

In terms of which milk to drink, organic goat's milk is probably the most health-promoting option. If you find it too expensive or unpalatable or inaccessible, at the very least choose whole-fat dairy products for your family — they'll thank you for it.

5

READING
INGREDIENTS

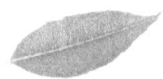

Years ago, when my oldest was little and the days were hot, I bought my kids popsicles that I thought contained natural ingredients because the label read, "No food coloring," which temporarily put me at ease. After tasting one, I commented to my husband, "This tastes just like those artificial punch drinks they used to give us in camp!" We looked back at the package and, lo and behold, no coloring, but yes artificial flavors and preservatives (sulfites). Oh well...

After that, I became more cautious when purchasing packaged foods. Often, you can learn a lot more from what is *not* said. If the package advertises, "No preservatives," it probably contains coloring or flavors. "Flavors" usually means artificial flavors. Even if the package states, "All natural ingredients," I recommend you read the details for yourself to see if your definition of "all natural" is the same as the manufacturer's. But if you really want to know what you are eating, make homemade.

As a child, I was fascinated by the concept of food coloring. *Wow,* I thought, *it looks like a marker, but it's really food!* Later on, I was disenchanted when I discovered that most of those vivid "food-grade" shades were a lot closer to marker than food.

REAL CHOCOLATE?

I used to wonder why some chocolate chips say "real," while other, less-expensive, ones are missing the word. The answer is really quite simple if you put the packages side by side and compare ingredients. Both usually contain sugar and cocoa mass, but the next ingredient is where the two part ways; real chocolate contains naturally occurring cocoa butter, while "fake" chocolate contains hydrogenated fat instead.

HYDROGENATED FATS

Margarine and shortening are synthetic fats, created in a laboratory. They were invented to replace animal fats like butter (and lard), since animal fats are high in cholesterol and saturated fat, which were erroneously blamed for heart disease. Margarine and shortening contain no cholesterol, which is only found in animal products, and are low in saturated fats and high in *hydrogenated* polyunsaturated fats.

It was alleged that margarine could be used to reduce cholesterol and saturated fat intake and thereby improve vascular (circulatory/heart) health. Time has proven that these theories were totally off the mark. To the dismay of avid margarine users, hydrogenated fats are more likely to *increase* the incidence of heart attack and even cancer. Watch out, since there are margarines that are sold as "natural" but contain hydrogenated fats.[37] [38]

One large-scale study on the effect of diet on fertility in 18,000 women found that **of all foods tested, trans fats were the most damaging** to fertility. As little as four grams a day (two tablespoons) was enough to have a detrimental effect.[39]

---

37   Mary G. Enig, *Know Your Fats: The Complete Primer for Understanding the Nutrition of Fats, Oil and Cholesterol*, 2000.

38   M. Enig, S.F. Morell, *The Oiling of America*, 2000, Weston Price Foundation.

39   M.D. Willett, Jorge E. Chavarro, C. Walter; Patrick Skerrett, "Fat, Carbs and the Science of Conception," *Newsweek*, Harmon Newsweek LLC. 2007.

PALM KERNEL OIL

In response to the public outcry and legislation against trans fats in the US, food manufacturers began using polyunsaturated vegetable oils, like sunflower and canola — a very bad idea, since these oils are unstable and are denatured (i.e., spoiled) when heated. They have also begun using palm kernel oil instead. This is definitely a major improvement over hydrogenated fats. Similar to coconut oil, palm kernel is very high in naturally occurring saturated fats, which makes it very stable. It has a long shelf life and can tolerate very high heat.

When you are grocery shopping, read labels and choose foods with high-quality ingredients. The more demand there is for genuine natural foods, the more they will become available to consumers.

6

FLUORIDE

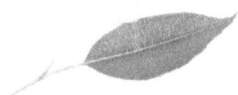

Fluoride is found in nearly every tube of toothpaste. In many areas, it is also added to public water supply. Recently, there has been an increased interest in fluoride-free toothpaste. Additionally, while most US cities fluoridate their water, most of Western Europe has banned or rejected water fluoridation for the most part, due to safety concerns.[40]

The following statement appeared on the back of a fluoride-free toothpaste in our medicine cabinet:

> "Some people do not want fluoride in their toothpaste. We produce this toothpaste without fluoride because we respect our customers' diverse needs and interests."

"Diverse needs and interests?" Why does this manufacturer use such bizarre language to describe the rejection of fluoride by some of their customers? My guess is that since this company makes another toothpaste *with* fluoride, they won't come out and tell you that fluoride

---

40   Fluoride Action Network, "Statements from European Health, Water, & Environment Authorities on Water Fluoridation," 2007.

is harmful, only that some unusual people suffer from an idiosyncrasy that causes them to prefer fluoride-free for no apparent reason...

THE HYGIENIST

A few years ago, my son came home from school with a toothbrush and a small tube of toothpaste. "A dental hygienist came to our class today," he announced. "She told us to brush our teeth at least twice a day. But she said to be very careful with the toothpaste, because it has fluoride in it, and if a kid would, *chas v'shalom* (G-d forbid), swallow everything in the tube, he could be *niftar* (killed)!"

And they are just handing this stuff out to little boys and trusting them to be responsible with it? I wondered to myself. "If this toothpaste is that unsafe, I do not want to have it in the house," I told my son. He was agreeable and threw the tube in the garbage. (More recently, I have started storing fluoride toothpaste that finds its way into our home out of reach, with the ant poison. I've been doing that since my nephew informed me that toothpaste can be used to seal ant holes. Apparently, ants don't like toothpaste. Is it the fluoride they are avoiding? I have yet to do a comparative study, but this is now our family's only use for fluoride toothpaste.)

SAFE BECAUSE IT'S…AVAILABLE?

We are told that fluoride prevents tooth decay, but is only safe in small quantities. Large amounts of fluoride toothpaste can be deadly, and yet we give the sweetened minty (or bubblegum flavored!) stuff to our kids and hope they don't swallow any of it. Is it really worth the risk, giving our children (and ourselves) a little bit of poison to prevent tooth decay?

In the past, I picked up products at the pharmacy (such as spray antiperspirant) and wondered, *Is this stuff really safe?* Then I answered myself, *It must be, or they wouldn't be selling it.* Since then, I've done a lot more research and have discovered that widespread use of a product, or even FDA approval, is **no** assurance of safety.

Now let's play a game. Try to guess the answers in the following True or False statements before reading further.

FLUORIDE TRUE OR FALSE

1. Fluoride is a deadly poison.
2. Fluoride prevents cavities and tooth decay, and rigorous, scientifically sound studies were conducted, proving fluoride effective.
3. Fluoride is an industrial toxic waste.
4. Primitive populations have always had terrible teeth.
5. Thanks to fluoride, Westerners have excellent teeth with no tooth decay.
6. Yearly fluoride rinses are an important way to prevent tooth decay.

Now let's consider these one by one.

1. Fluoride is a deadly poison.

True. Even the toothpaste manufacturers acknowledge this well-known fact. However, convoluted logic is used to explain the presence of toxic substances in our toiletries and pharmaceuticals. All too many times, I have heard the following mind-numbing argument: "All substances are deadly, given the right dose. Even too much water can kill a person...The amounts of [fluoride, aluminum, mercury, arsenic, lead, etc.] being used are so small that there is no danger."

This logic is highly flawed. Why? Because while ridiculously huge quantities of water may kill a person, water is not a poison. A poison is a substance that is dangerous or deadly even in small amounts. "An average-weighing two-year-old child could die from ingesting just forty percent of a Colgate for Kids bubble-gum flavored toothpaste."[41]

Additionally, many poisons are deadly in large amounts, while even tiny (microgram) quantities of these same substances can cause chronic damage.[42] **No** amount of fluoride is healthy or safe for human consumption. Chronic low-dose exposure to fluoride causes it to build up in the body (the bones).

---

41 Michael Connett, "The Minimum Lethal Dose of Fluoride," April 2012, http://fluoridealert.org/studies/acute01/.

42 Nancy Trautmann, "The Dose Makes the Poison — Or Does It?" *Bioscience* 2005, American Institute of Biological Sciences.

Industry and government have long had a powerful motive for claiming that fluoride is safe. But maintaining this position has not been easy since fluoride is one of the most toxic substances known... Evidence that industrial fluoride has been killing and crippling human beings has existed at least since the 1930s.[43]

2. Fluoride prevents cavities and tooth decay, and rigorous, scientifically sound studies were conducted, proving fluoride effective.

False. Based on the (mistaken) belief that fluoride strengthens the bones, clinical trials were conducted using fluoride to treat osteoporosis. The results were increased fractures, even in the absence of traumatic injury![44] It was found that fluoride *worsened* osteoporosis. How? Fluoride causes lead (a notoriously toxic metal) to *displace* calcium in the bones.[45] This means that it pushes calcium *out* of the bones, which causes bones to become brittle. After these catastrophic results, attempts at using fluoride to treat osteoporosis have been discontinued.

Have you ever heard of dental fluorosis? Believe it or not, this is a well-documented condition where teeth develop staining and pitting, due to...fluoride exposure. Even the World Health Organization describes dental and skeletal fluorosis, but continues to defend small doses as effective against tooth decay, claiming that this unwanted effect is only the result of overdose (in drinking water!).[46] Fluoride is so corrosive that it can actually bore holes through your water filter (and, of course, your teeth), making water filters in areas with fluoridated water ineffective after a few weeks. *Could fluoride really prevent cavities while the same substance has been proven to be corrosive to teeth and bones?*

---

43 Joel Griffiths, "Fluoride: Industry's Toxic Coup," *Food & Water Journal*, 1998.

44 Michael Connett, "Clinical Trials: Fluoride Treatment and Bone Fracture in Osteoporosis Patients," Fluoride Action Network, April 2012.

45 Russel L. Blaylock, MD, *Health and Nutrition Secrets That Can Save Your Life*, Health Press, 2006.

46 World Health Organization, "Water-related diseases," http://www.who.int/water_sanitation_health/diseases/fluorosis/en/.

How fluoride gained its reputation for preventing cavities:

> In 1931, a PHS (US Public Health Service) dentist named H. Trendley Dean was dispatched to remote towns in the West where drinking-water wells contained high concentrations of natural fluoride. His mission: to determine how much fluoride people could tolerate without sustaining obvious damage to their teeth. Dean found that teeth in these high-fluoride towns were often discolored and eroded, but he also reported that they appeared to have fewer cavities than average.[47]

And that was the basis for fluoride's use in dental care. Assuming that Dr. Dean's conclusions about cavity prevention were accurate (which seems unlikely, considering the contradictory findings), a very strange picture emerges: Fluoride corrodes and stains teeth, and yet should be added to water *to improve dental health*? The same substance that has been proven to corrode teeth is being used to *protect* them...

3. Fluoride is an industrial toxic waste.

True. Fluoride is a by-product of aluminum manufacturing. Incredibly toxic, manufacturers were obliged to spend a fortune to safely dispose of fluoride. That is, until it gained the weakly supported reputation for preventing tooth decay. Now, instead of wasting hard-earned industry money to dispose of it, industrial manufacturers can conveniently *sell* their toxic waste to water suppliers, dentists, and toothpaste manufacturers.

In the 1930s, "The University of Cincinnati's Kettering Laboratory, funded largely by top fluoride emitters such as Alcoa (The Aluminum Company of America), quickly dominated fluoride-safety research. A book by Kettering scientist (and Reynolds Metals consultant) E.J. Largent was admittedly written in part to 'aid industry in lawsuits arising from fluoride damage.' Nonetheless, the book became a basic

---

47   Joel Griffiths, "Fluoride: Industry's Toxic Coup." *Food & Water Journal*, Summer 1998.

international reference work"[48] used to prove the effectiveness of fluoride for preventing dental carries (i.e., cavities).

4. Primitive populations have always had terrible teeth.

False. For centuries, many non-Westernized populations the world over had nearly perfect teeth. This phenomenon was studied in great depth by Dr. Weston Price, a dentist who traveled the world in search of populations with little tooth decay, to determine which dietary and lifestyle habits prevented it.

What he discovered was that on many varying traditional diets, teeth, bone structure, and overall health were excellent. When these populations switched over to the "white" Western diet, containing mostly white flour, white sugar, and preserves, tooth decay, birth defects, bone malformation, and disease became rampant.

Though most of us (including myself) have long believed that primitive populations like the Australian Aborigines and the Native Americans were decimated due to exposure to the new germs that the Europeans introduced, this may not have been the foremost source of their destruction. It would seem that it was the malnutrition the natives experienced when they first encountered and traded for the "white man's" foods that ultimately made them vulnerable to contagious disease. The Western diet brought malnutrition and death to *many* populations.[49]

Bottom line: A high-sugar diet is the ultimate source of tooth decay, but for a different reason than most people believe. It is because sugar causes malnutrition, and malnutrition weakens the teeth, which makes them susceptible to decay. Primitive populations had no sugar, and when they ate according to their ancient traditional diets, they had straight and perfect teeth.

At the dentist last week, I lamented that I try so hard to give my kids a sound and healthy diet, and yet they still develop cavities! "What do you expect?" he responded. "We're living in Candy Land!" What

---

48   Ibid.

49   Weston A. Price, DDS, *Nutrition and Physical Degeneration*, 8th edition, Price-Pottenger Nutrition Foundation, 1939–2014.

an accurate description. From their first year in playgroup, the sweet incentives begin... And there is no end in sight.

5. Thanks to fluoride, Westerners have excellent teeth with no tooth decay.

False. Look around you; most kids today have a mouth full of cavities. Tooth decay is *rampant* in Western civilization, and fluoride has done nothing to stem the tide. The real way to prevent tooth decay is from the inside out. Sugar does not merely feed bacteria in the mouth. This is a misconception. The real problem with sugar is that too much of it causes malnutrition. The way to prevent cavities and tooth decay is with proper nutrition that provides for strong teeth and bones.[50] Fluoride weakens teeth and bones and causes loss of essential minerals.[51]

6. Yearly fluoride rinses are an important way to prevent tooth decay.

False. An acquaintance of mine who is well-informed about health took her kids to the dentist for a checkup. The hygienist told her that it was time for their yearly fluoride rinse. "No, thanks," she responded. The hygienist was shocked. Nobody refuses (insurance-covered) dental procedures! The dentist stormed in and angrily threatened the mother that her children would suffer from devastating tooth decay. She would not be swayed, because she had already researched the subject and knew that they were wrong. They noted in their charts that she was "noncompliant." While small amounts of fluoride may or may not have dire health consequences in the long run, the amounts used in fluoride rinses contradict even their own logic that fluoride need not be feared since the doses are so minute.

Finally, don't feel bad to throw out a tube of fluoridated toothpaste. It's worth every penny. Look for fluoride-free options and experiment until you find the product that works best for you. Many people have asked me which toothpaste I recommend. There is no one-size-fits-all answer. People will respond differently to the same products. Just be an educated consumer, and read the ingredients before you purchase.

---

50   Ibid.
51   Russel L. Blaylock, MD, *Health and Nutrition Secrets That Can Save Your Life*, Health Press, 2006.

7

WATER

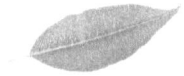

One winter, a patient came to me complaining of muscle pain and lethargy. Among other things, I asked her about her fluid consumption, and she told me that she drank at least eight to ten cups of water a day. After evaluating her constitution, I recommended that she try *reducing* her fluid intake. I suggested that she try to become more aware of her body's cues and drink when she felt she needed to, and stop drinking when she felt she'd had enough.

The following week, she reported excitedly that after following my advice and reducing fluid intake, her body felt lighter and more energetic. She also realized that while abiding by her previous regimen of eight to ten cups of water, her digestion was sluggish, and she felt bloated constantly.

We always hear that water flushes out and cleanses the body, and therefore the more the better. In reality, the kidneys have to work to flush water out of our system, so overconsumption can actually be quite taxing.

A standardized, one-size-fits-all fluid-volume recommendation does not make much sense when you take into account the wide variety of physical constitutions. Different people need different amounts of water. Also, the body's needs change depending on the season. Most people do not need the same amount of fluids in the winter as they do in the summer. In a dry environment, you will need to drink more than you would in a humid climate. While not drinking enough gets a lot of attention, drinking too much can be equally unhealthy! Listen to your body's cues and drink when you feel thirsty.

That being said, we are all different. Some individuals never experience thirst. While lack of thirst may be a sign of your body's needs, there are people who become dehydrated because they never get the thirst message. The key here is that if you never feel thirsty but tend to experience symptoms of dehydration (headaches, dizziness, nausea, abdominal pain, fatigue, etc.) then you should probably not rely on your body's cues for hydration needs.

Often, patients tell me that they drink tons of fluids but then find themselves running to the bathroom immediately afterward. If this is the case, what they are drinking is not being absorbed at all! Ironically, these people may absorb fluids better by drinking less. Even if you are very thirsty, it is better to drink small amounts frequently than guzzle a large amount all at once.

Some people find that they do not absorb plain water well. If that happens to you, you may benefit from adding one or more of the following to your water: a pinch of pink Himalayan salt, a pinch of baking soda, a squeeze of lemon, or a small amount of apple cider vinegar. The Rambam (Maimonides) advises against drinking during meals and recommends waiting until after to drink. If you are very thirsty and must drink during your meal, he advises adding a bit of wine to your water when you drink during a meal.

Some people tolerate tea or other beverages better than water. To differentiate between healthy messages from your body and unhealthy cravings, consider how you feel *after* the drink. Not just immediately after, but even an hour or two later. Sugary or caffeinated drinks give a very transient energy boost that is usually followed by a crash, leaving one weaker than they were before the sugary beverage.

Too much fruit juice is rarely a good idea, specifically orange juice, which has developed a reputation for being "packed" with vitamin C and has therefore been alleged to ward off the common cold. There are three problems with orange juice, all of which make it a liability rather than an asset for your immune system:

1. Orange juice is full of rapidly absorbed sugar (think high glycemic index/"fast" carb). High sugar levels actually deplete vitamin C stores in the body.
2. Orange juice produces a lot of mucus in the body, which is the opposite of what one would need when fighting or trying to prevent a cold.
3. And this is the clincher: the claim that orange juice contains the 100 percent daily value of vitamin C is bogus. The amount of vitamin C in most juices is closer to 0 mg.

Why does orange juice contain so little vitamin C? Vitamin C is very sensitive and rapidly deteriorates upon exposure to heat, air, and light. The process of juicing and heat pasteurization will destroy most, if not all, the vitamin C from the orange. Also, even with the remote possibility that the package is telling you the truth and the juice really *does* contain 60 mg of vitamin C per serving, most people need somewhere between 1000 and 5000 mg per day to maintain health! (See chapter on vitamin C for more information.)

Drinking excessive quantities of orange juice can cause more harm than good. Aside from mucus production, orange juice can exacerbate hyperactivity, eczema, and asthma. When foods cause exhaustion, headaches, mood changes, or mucus production, you should probably limit intake of that food.

What we can learn from oranges is that we can't just look at the nutritional content on the food label. We also must look at how the food interacts with our body. This is also true for water consumption. If you feel weighed down and bloated, you may need to change your drinking habits. Hopefully, once you become aware of your body's needs, you will be able to improve your family's health with your own intuition.

8

ICE

AND INJURIES

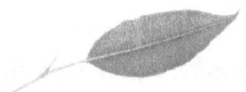

A patient once came to me for treatment of a fracture that had occurred over a year earlier. X-rays showed that the injury had healed, but she was still experiencing severe pain and swelling. Her doctors advised her to continue icing the area (which she had been doing since she began rehabilitation). Meanwhile, she was taking painkillers daily. It seemed that the healing process had come to a grinding halt, with no explanation.

The first thing I told her was to stop icing — permanently. She responded excitedly, "Since I got the injury, I hated icing it — I found it excruciating! I only continued to do it because of my doctor's insistence. I really felt like it was doing more harm than good!"

Her instincts were right. We have become so accustomed to icing our injuries that we may be ignoring clear messages from our body. The burning, numbness, and pain we feel with ice is purportedly part of the healing process. Ice is used to bring down swelling. As long as this goal is even temporarily achieved, we are satisfied. Since swelling is bad, ice must be good. But what happens after the swelling comes down? Will the injury heal? Sometimes. But that is not because of the ice, but in spite of it. As we shall see, there is more to the healing process than instant results.

Let us look at the nature of ice. Freezing water transforms it from a free-flowing state to one of stillness. So if ice is still, what does it do to the body? Since the freezing process slows down the movement of fluids, ice will do the same thing to the body; it will slow the flow of blood through the injured area. In order for the healing process to progress, we need circulation to be free and smooth. Ice prevents that. So what happens to the healing process when an injury is iced? It is halted.

Back to the patient above: When I felt her ankle, I was not surprised to discover that the swollen area was quite cold to the touch. The ice had caused "coldness" to lodge itself in her ankle. I gave her acupuncture to promote better circulation through the area. Then, I wrote her a prescription for a warming herbal soak to counteract the effects of the ice and restart the healing process.

We may have assumed that the cold lasts only as long as the ice remains on the body. But in truth, even temporary exposure to cold can leave a long-lasting negative imprint. This is especially so if ice is used repeatedly. People with arthritic conditions can often detect weather changes. They can feel the cold, damp weather in their bones. Cold weather is often the instigator for arthritic conditions. Using ice on arthritic joints can exacerbate the problem, even if it gives temporary relief.

OTHER OPTIONS

Ice has always been the only recourse for the treatment of injuries at home. Is there anything else we can do?

- Immediately after mild injury, it is beneficial to massage the area; this will increase the blood flow and accelerate healing. Even a light rub can go a long way. Isn't that what we do instinctively in response to injury?
- For muscle aches, especially those that feel cold to the touch, try hot-water bottles, heating pads, or a hot bath.

- Not all injuries are cold. Sometimes they are red and quite warm to the touch. Even in these cases, ice will not be beneficial in the long run, but will prolong the healing process. A better option is to use a cooling herbal soak or ointment (such as one containing menthol) that is applied at room temperature.

Children are masters of injury; they are constantly banging one part of their body or another. When this happens, our first (and usually only) recourse is to get some sort of frozen item and hold it there until the child's screaming (if he is too young to understand that the ice is supposed to be helping) becomes unbearable.

Try simply rubbing the boo-boo instead. You will find that not only will this usually calm and comfort the recently traumatized child far more quickly than ice will, but it will also help to reduce bruising and pain in the area — starting immediately. You will not be disappointed. And next time someone bangs their head, keep that freezer door closed!

9

HERBAL
MEDICINE

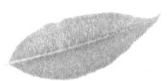

W hile I was studying Chinese medicine, a number of my relatives were diagnosed with high cholesterol. At the time, I was not the avid researcher that I am today, so I took it for granted that high cholesterol was a real disease that warranted treatment. I heard from one of my fellow classmates that the original source of Lipitor was a plant from China called red yeast rice. It is actually more fungus than rice. Based on my colleague's recommendation, I told all my relatives about red yeast rice as a natural cholesterol-lowering alternative, and everyone was happy to try it.

It wasn't long before the complaints started rolling in. Red yeast rice was causing terrible stomach pain and other ill effects. Disappointed, all three of my relatives eventually discontinued using it. It was only many years later that I was to finally understand what had gone so wrong with their "natural" treatment of an otherwise symptomless disease known as hypercholesteremia.

There are many plants, some of which are used medicinally, that can be poisonous and even deadly. Not everything nature has to offer is safe.

The concept of using small amounts of poisons medicinally is as old as time. Some things are labeled "natural" because they come directly from nature, and yet are still poisonous and cannot be considered safe.

Some things that are natural are also deadly poisons, including many mushrooms, arsenic, and heavy metals like mercury and aluminum. Even in their purest natural form they are deadly. The word "natural" can actually be a convenient way for product manufacturers to hide dangerous ingredients in plain sight, since they can be found in nature. Manufacturers can include something as deadly as mercury in their product and label it deceptively as "all natural"!

Some plants have no medicinal use. Some have been altered in a way that causes them to impart dangerous effects on the body that cannot be considered medicinal. One example of an unsafe and useless "natural remedy" is the popular modern-day version of red yeast rice; animals that eat this plant in large quantities can be killed by it. Scientists discovered that this plant blocks cholesterol production and it became the basis for statin drugs. People who want to go natural and use red yeast rice instead of Lipitor often find that it causes as many or more side effects than the drug itself!

The ability of red yeast rice to block cholesterol production is what makes it so dangerous. Interestingly, red yeast rice was not in common use in traditional Chinese medicine. It was only *after* pharmaceutical companies used it to manufacture Lipitor that people went "back to nature" for the original, and the product then became insanely popular. Using red yeast rice to block cholesterol production is as dangerous as taking statin drugs.

Many herbs cannot be used during pregnancy or while nursing. Well-trained herbalists are very cautious about prescribing herbs to pregnant women, and should be well aware of which herbs can be safely used during this time period.

Aside from pregnancy, most medicinal herbs are usually only harmful when taken in excessive doses. This situation can be avoided by following the age-old prescribing rules. Every competent herbalist is well versed in the safe dosage of herbs.

Still, herbs can be rendered unsafe when they are concentrated into pharmaceutical products to make them more potent. Some plant-based pharmaceuticals use herbs in unprecedented high doses. The potential for problems is enormous.

The caution exercised when using herbs and supplements should be applied to pharmaceuticals as well. "Something is very wrong when regulatory agencies pretend that vitamins are dangerous, yet ignore published statistics showing that government-sanctioned medicine is the real hazard."[52]

In the US, the total number of deaths caused by conventional medicine has reached 783,936 per year. **Shockingly, modern medicine is now the leading cause of death,** followed by heart disease and cancer. Of these deaths, **106,000 per year** are caused by adverse drug reactions. This includes drugs taken correctly in normal dosage range.

To put things in perspective, let us take a look at the most potent and lethal Chinese herb: aconite. In China, over a period of thirty years, six hundred people were reported to have suffered from aconite poisoning due to incorrect preparation of the herb and patient-prescribed overdose. Compare this to acetaminophen (Tylenol), which the FDA links to nearly one thousand deaths per year.[53]

When used correctly, medicine should not produce any side effects. This does not mean that it is incapable of doing so. It means that if side effects occur, it's a sign that this is not the right remedy. I know that I've prescribed correctly if my patient feels better, not worse *in any way*, giving an adjustment period of a few days at the onset of a new treatment.

On the rare occasion that patients experience ongoing side effects from herbs (stomachache being the most common, in my experience), I advise them to discontinue their herbal treatment immediately. I certainly do not think side effects from herbs are impossible, but they *are* unacceptable. When it comes to medicine, I believe that something cannot make you healthier if it simultaneously makes you sicker. Even

52   Gary Null, PhD, Carolyn Dean, MD, ND, Martin Feldman, MD, Debora Rasio, MD, and Dorothy Smith, PhD, "Death by Medicine," lef.org.

53   T.C. Miller, Jeff Gerth, "Behind the Numbers," Propublica.org/article/Tylenol-mcneil-fda-behind-the-numbers, Sept. 20, 2013.

if blood tests show improvement, if the patient feels worse, it's not a good sign.

Certain medical treatments can cause a temporary worsening of symptoms, which is then followed by improvement. This happens occasionally in patients who receive acupuncture for a pain condition. I warn my patients that sometimes it may feel worse before it gets better. There is a special acupuncture treatment I particularly like to use that has the effect of producing an emotional release. Sometimes this comes out as anger, but this is very short-lived and followed by a period of genuine emotional improvement.

When I treat babies for constipation using acupuncture, sometimes they can be grouchy for a day or two after the treatment before the bowels start to move. The treatment can cause some initial discomfort, but after that, when it works, the relief ensues.

Some detoxification programs (not something I personally use in my practice, so I cannot vouch for it clinically) that use juicing or fasting or other forms of detoxification, prepare their patients for what some call a "healing crisis," which is defined as the point when the body starts to release toxins. It can cause flu-like symptoms, headaches, changes in bowel or urine, or other strange symptoms. If this is truly beneficial, it should soon be followed by improvement in energy and overall well-being. Any serious detoxification program should be conducted under the supervision of a healthcare practitioner experienced in this area.

The bottom line is that if side effects are possible in a given treatment, it's best to know about them in advance, be prepared for them, and understand whether they are a sign that the treatment is harming the person or will pass and leave them in better health. If the side effects last longer than two weeks, it's time to start questioning the treatment.

One of my greatest frustrations, which I see so often in my clinic, is that many people are suffering from side effects of drugs without anyone realizing that the source of their new and chronic condition is the medication they are taking. So while short-term negative effects may be acceptable as a part of healing, long-term side effects indicate that the treatment is creating new health problems.

At the end of the day, it is a matter of choice. Some people choose to accept the side effects of their medications, hoping that the benefits outweigh the harm. Others reject medicine that makes them ill and instead pursue treatments that make them feel better and healthier overall.

After my articles are published in magazines, we often receive letters. I have included them throughout the book where they relate to the topic at hand.[54] While my articles induce plenty of positive feedback, those letters are not nearly as interesting and therefore they are rarely included.

> *Dear Editor,*
>
> *I'd like to quote you Yael Tusk's article. "In the US, the total number of deaths caused by conventional medicine has reached 783,936 per year." Fewer people were harmed by alternative medicine because fewer were treated.*
>
> *And please don't bring me any figures from China. Don't even try to compare their record keeping to Western records. If 600 deaths were reported over 30 years, that really scares me; it could be the real numbers are 60,000, who knows?*
>
> *Besides, if we're talking about people overdosing, if they had the Chinese herbs available, they would have overdosed on them. This is the exact problem with alternative medicine — it is not exact (or, at least, not as exact as Western medicine), and don't pretend that it's an exact science that can replace modern medicine.*
>
> *Please don't misunderstand me. Alternative medicine has its place. In fact, I'm taking my son to a chiropractor. But it's ALTERNATIVE, meaning that our main medical treatments are by the doctors who have*

---

54   Letters may be edited or summarized.

proven themselves to deliver safe and effective medicines. Western medicine eradicated many fatal diseases and has significantly increased the life expectancy of worldwide humanity. Please do not undermine it and, especially, do not doubt the effectiveness and safety of the vaccinations that have saved many lives.

Although it has its place, alternative medicine has yet to prove itself effective enough to replace Western medicine.

M.C.

This was my response to the letter-writer:

Dear M.C.,

If you feel confident in the safety of modern medicine despite the fact that it is killing more people in the US each year than the leading deadly diseases (cancer and heart disease), that is certainly your prerogative.

To be conservative, let us suppose that only ten percent of US citizens utilize alternative medicine on a regular basis. If alternative medicine caused as much devastation as modern medicine, we would expect to see roughly 78,393 deaths every year from holistic medicine. Do we? Not even close!

The lack of systematic regulation of alternative medicine has not resulted in huge numbers of death or injury. The reason that herbal medicine has never been rigorously controlled in the same fashion that modern medicine is, is because most herbs are not inherently dangerous. While, of course, there are herbs that can be harmful when abused or used in excessive doses, this still remains a rare occurrence. Herbs and drugs are inherently different. Herbs are inherently safe in almost all cases, while pharmaceutical drugs are inherently unsafe, no matter how heavily regulated.

Chinese herbal medicine has a clear-cut safe dosage range for every single herb. This is well-established scientifically. The amount of herbs needed to reach a lethal dose is far higher than most pharmaceuticals, where often one bottle of pills may be enough to kill a person.

The fact that everything outside the framework of Western medicine has been labeled "alternative" is the work of modern medicine alone. There is no real reason that all forms of holistic medicine have been relegated outside the camp. In terms of effectiveness and safety, many forms of natural medicine are a real force to be reckoned with — and have thousands of years of history, experience, and healthy societies on their side.

Is the modern medical infrastructure that is intended to filter out good from bad science, such as FDA approval and peer-reviewed studies, enough to ensure the safety of its consumers? Does FDA approval render a drug safe? Western medicine has certainly become very technologically advanced and is capable of saving lives, particularly in the area of emergency medicine. Still, a look at history and an evaluation of various successes and failures in medicine reveals a much more complicated picture. Invasive medicine and artificial drugs cause an enormous amount of serious problems, and are less successful than we may expect them to be.

Regarding safety, conventional medicine as it is practiced today cannot be rendered safe through regulation alone. When working with something that is inherently dangerous, as is the case with many pharmaceutical drugs as well as most surgical procedures, the risks remain despite rigorous oversight.

I recently heard a quote from someone who said, "While modern medicine may kill people with its powerful yet deadly treatments, alternative medicine kills more people due to its lack of effectiveness." Even if they were right in their presumption that all forms of holistic medicine are worthless (they're not), they would be hardpressed to explain how a medicine that is not deadly could be capable of killing more people than a medicine that actively kills around a million people a year in the US alone.

10

CHOLESTEROL

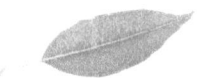

I have heard many versions of the following story over the years: A number of years ago, Rita was diagnosed with high cholesterol. She was told that her liver was malfunctioning. Her doctor advised her to avoid foods with lots of cholesterol (meat, dairy, eggs...). That didn't help her, and she was then told that her body was *producing* too much cholesterol. It had nothing to do with how much she was eating, because her foolish liver just kept on pumping out those stubborn lipoproteins.

She was then prescribed Lipitor (a statin drug that blocks cholesterol production). Rita is one of several million who has received this diagnosis. According to the ever-decreasing threshold for healthy cholesterol levels, around sixty percent of adults over sixty-five are being diagnosed with high cholesterol and prescribed statins![55]

STATINS AND MEMORY LOSS

Very soon after starting on Lipitor, Rita's memory started failing her. She heard from friends that this might be a side effect of the Lipitor, so

---

55 Kowa Pharmaceuticals America, Statin Usage, http://www.statinusage.com/Pages/choles-terol-overview.aspx, 2013.

she did the responsible thing and asked her doctor. He told her that he had never heard of a connection between statins and memory loss.

Trusting her doctor's knowledge of the risks of a drug that he was prescribing, she continued to take her medication loyally for many more years. All the while, her memory has continued to deteriorate.

HEART DISEASE IN CHICKS?

Did you ever wonder why chicks (baby chickens) do not hatch with terrible circulatory problems, considering that they are nourished on incredibly high levels of cholesterol from the yolk sack before they hatch? There's an explanation for why their hearts are fine: Experts explain that they now realize that there are two types of cholesterol — HDL and LDL (high- and low-density lipoprotein). LDL has been labeled "bad," and HDL, the "good" cholesterol.

Chicks aren't born nearly dead from cholesterol toxicity because they are nourished with lots of the "good" cholesterol before they hatch. The result of separating lipoproteins into high- and low-density is that eggs are no longer considered a danger to the heart. They have become "heart healthy" once again. Doctors who stay up-to-date are now encouraging their patients to start eating eggs again! This was happy news for many egg fans and many sufferers of the infamous "egg-white omelet."

There is something very strange going on here. Let's establish some facts. **HDL and LDL are not cholesterol**. Think of them as little vehicles that *carry* cholesterol and fat through the bloodstream. The only difference between these carriers is their size and the concentration of the nutrients within them.

You read that correctly: cholesterol is a nutrient. It is an essential component of all cellular function, and is found in remarkably high levels in the healthy human brain There is only one type of cholesterol. However, according to current medical beliefs, when cholesterol is transported by LDLs, it's bad for you. But when you put the same substance in a smaller package (HDL), it is now (very) good for you.

What does the world look like when your eyes are closed?

Rita's doctor was not aware of a connection between Lipitor and memory loss, and was therefore unable to recognize the side effect his patient was suffering from.

The fact is, though, it does not take much effort to unearth the abundant evidence connecting statins with memory loss. There is even a clear pathological mechanism that explains why this happens. Our livers are not producing cholesterol by accident; cholesterol is needed for *all* cellular functions.

A whopping twenty-five percent of your body's cholesterol is found in the brain, keeping neurons connected and helping with all levels of brain function. Drastically reduce your body's cholesterol supply, and your brain will be the first to suffer. This is a vast oversimplification, but you get the idea.

Isn't cholesterol causing heart disease?

There is ample evidence that cholesterol does not cause heart disease. In fact, blocking our liver's ability to produce cholesterol (the mechanism of statin drugs, such as Lipitor) can have dire health consequences.

When an article I wrote on this subject appeared in a magazine, we received the following letter from a reader:

> *Dear Editor,*
>
> *I am a physical organic chemist, and Yael Tusk's cholesterol article has prompted me to respond... She mentions that her client heard from friends that statins might cause memory loss. The client asked her doctor, who had never heard of the connection. I checked the insert included with each prescription. Memory loss and confusion are mentioned three separate times. The problem is with the doctor and not the pharmaceutical information. At least 35 million people in the world today have dementia. I know many people who are affected, and most were nowhere near statins!*
>
> *High-density lipoproteins are considered good carriers because, unlike low-density lipoproteins, they, so to speak, do not get caught in the arteries and cause*

plaque. The plaques are not solely cholesterol, but that is another topic.

I would hope that the doctors' pledge would also apply to Yael: "First do no harm." The health of her readers may depend on her words.

Sophia

This was my response to the letter-writer:

Dear Sophia,

While the body can produce harmful substances, it can only cause damage to itself if something has gone awry. Hydrochloric acid is a dangerous substance if it is found outside the stomach. However, in the stomach it acts as a digestive aid and a crucial first line of immune defense, neutralizing potentially dangerous microorganisms.

Cholesterol is not a harmful substance. It does not cause heart disease. I have seen innumerable patients who were suffering from side effects from their medications. When they asked their doctors, they were told that their new symptoms were unrelated to the prescriptions they were taking. This was despite the fact that drug inserts often listed the very side effects that they were experiencing. Package inserts are rarely given enough attention before starting on medication. I encourage everyone to read package inserts thoroughly and carefully before initiating any medication.

Pharmaceutical companies acknowledge that drugs that reduce cholesterol can cause memory loss and confusion. Does this fact make cognitive deterioration acceptable? Should it occur? If someone taking statins begins to lose their memory, there may be other factors contributing to their memory loss (such as an overload of mercury or aluminum in the brain). It may, however, be the statins causing the problem, as the package insert warns. It is also possible that memory may improve if statins are abandoned.

For our entire lives, most of us have been convinced that cholesterol is a disease-causing substance. It can be difficult to see it any other way. As Mark Twain so aptly put it, "It's easier to fool people than to convince people that they've been fooled."

Hippocrates's "first do no harm" can be perfectly applied to statins. If they can cause dementia, diabetes, as well as many other possible side effects, is it justifiable to prescribe them — when safe, effective, and natural medicine exists? Drugs with such side effects are usually not necessary.

Some examples of effective forms of medicine that are low-risk:

- Acupuncture
- Herbal medicine — used within verified safe dosage range, and based on a long history of traditional use. Even safe herbs can be rendered dangerous when highly concentrated or abused. In fact, many pharmaceutical products have their roots in herbs. Morphine comes from poppy, a traditional Chinese herb. Nitroglycerin (which is actually a lifesaving remedy) has its roots in homeopathy!
- Homeopathic medicine
- Chiropractic
- Reflexology
- Craniosacral therapy
- Nutritional supplementation

Although all of these forms of healing have been labeled alternative and therefore relegated outside the mainstream camp, it is not because these methods are less effective, but simply because they are not part of the modern medical system. Most of these techniques are holistic, which means that they treat the body as a whole and work to improve overall health while treating the individual complaint.

If you are in excellent health and your only symptom is high cholesterol, then you need neither alternative nor modern medical treatment, because high cholesterol is actually no indication of illness. In fact, higher cholesterol levels may be protective against disease and may improve longevity![56]

---

56   Uffe Ravnskov, MD, PhD, "The Benefits of High Cholesterol," *The Cholesterol Myths* 12/30/2015 http://www.ravnskov.nu/2015/12/30/the-benefits-of-high-cholesterol/.

11

HEART
DISEASE

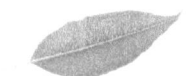

The cholesterol hypothesis is an ever-changing theory. Around the turn of the twentieth century, scientists were able to observe arterial plaques under the microscope. (Plaques thicken and clog the walls of arteries and are associated with coronary artery disease. Interestingly, plaques are only found in arteries, not veins.) They discovered that cholesterol was one of the main components in these plaques. Scientists concluded that cholesterol builds up on arterial walls and causes blockages. However, there were other components in those plaques, such as calcium and platelets, which were overlooked.

What if they'd noticed the calcium?

Despite the fact that calcium is present in arterial plaques, we have not been directed to minimize our dietary intake of calcium. Nor would anyone take calcium-reducing medication! This is because calcium has never been labeled as a cause of heart disease, even though it is found in the very same plaques that contain cholesterol. Just imagine if those early scientists had found the calcium in the plaques instead of cholesterol!

The fact that cholesterol is found in arterial plaques led to the mistaken notion that cholesterol is the *cause* of blockages. If this was true, then evidence would have shown a higher rate of heart disease in populations with higher cholesterol levels. Numerous studies have proven that this is not the case:[57]

According to Malcolm Kendrick, MD, the myth-busting researcher, and author of the groundbreaking book, *The Great Cholesterol Con*:

> The main man [to promote the diet heart hypotheses in the 1950s] was Ancel Keys and his famous Seven Countries Study. Keys looked at saturated-fat consumption in seven countries and found a straight-line relationship between heart disease, cholesterol level, and saturated fat intake.

The problem was that while these seven countries neatly proved his hypothesis, many countries that were not included in his analysis disproved it — countries like France, where dietary saturated fat and cholesterol intake is high, yet heart disease is low; and countries like Israel, where saturated fat and cholesterol consumption are low, yet heart-disease rates are high. When many countries' dietary intake and heart-disease rates are charted, the correlation disappears.[58]

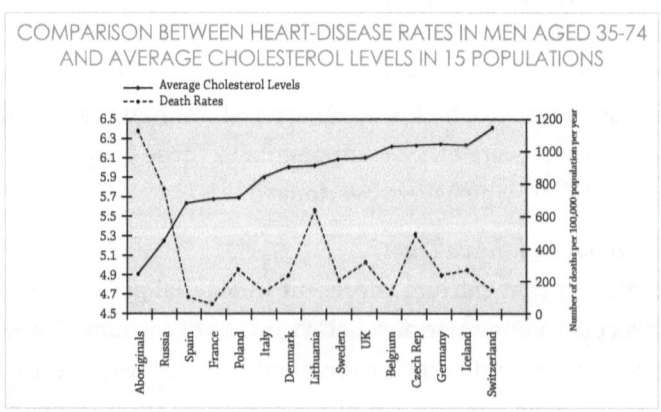

COMPARISON BETWEEN HEART-DISEASE RATES IN MEN AGED 35-74 AND AVERAGE CHOLESTEROL LEVELS IN 15 POPULATIONS

57   Kendrick, Malcolm, MD, *The Great Cholesterol Con*, 2007.
58   Ibid.

The above graph, which illustrates the findings of a World Health Organization study on trends in cardiovascular disease, clearly illustrates that there is no correlation between cholesterol and heart disease.

The theory that plaques form as a result of bulky cholesterol getting stuck en route was just that: a theory. While of course plaque accumulation *can* cause blockages and lead to heart attacks, they don't form at random, and have nothing to do with cholesterol level at all, as we shall soon see.

DAMAGED BLOOD VESSELS

Arterial plaques do not form at random — they form where there is arterial damage. The plaques act like bandages to seal damage to arterial walls. Every time there is damage in an arterial wall, the body uses calcium, cholesterol, platelets, and other components to repair that damage. Blood-vessel damage can lead to accumulation of plaque, which, when combined with blood clots, may eventually cause total blockage and can result in a full-blown heart attack. In other words, the plaques are not just an accidental accumulation of cholesterol, but the body's attempt to repair damaged tissue.

While many people don't like taking statins and are uncomfortable with the side effects — which commonly include muscle pain and atrophy, memory loss (both of which probably have something to do with cholesterol insufficiency), diabetes, liver damage, and kidney failure — at the same time, they fear that if they stop, their cholesterol levels will rise. In truth, should they go off their meds, their cholesterol probably will go up. But that's a good thing, because we need cholesterol, and there is no reason to fear a rising cholesterol level.

Statins are very effective in lowering cholesterol. They do so by blocking part of a very complex biochemical process in our liver's production of cholesterol. I would love to explain to you that process, but honestly, the makers of statins don't even really understand the process, though I am pretty certain that our Creator does. The liver is not producing cholesterol by accident. In almost all cases, the liver will produce exactly as much as cholesterol as the body needs. Blocking the body's natural cholesterol production can only cause harm.

Medical style varies greatly among doctors. Some doctors are terrific. Others seem to be on a hunt for illness, and no one can leave their offices without several prescriptions. A friend once complained that it's rare for her to go to her doctor without being told that something is wrong with her.

In my opinion, whenever these diagnoses affect an abnormally large portion of the population, there are a number of explanations:

1. **It's not a real disease**. High cholesterol is a good example of this. There is no plausible medical explanation for why or how the body is malfunctioning, except for some theoretical underlying defect. No pathology has been found that indicates that the liver's production of cholesterol is malfunctioning.

2. **Mankind is causing the problem**. Experience shows that the root cause of most genuine health problems is humanity's poor choices. Smoking, drugs, unhealthy food choices, overeating, radiation, pollution, unsafe medical procedures, poor hygiene, and poor nutrition are just a few examples of how we are hurting ourselves and each other. Indeed, this is probably our biggest health threat.

3. **Fate**. Sometimes we do the best we can but get sick nonetheless.

When we are presented with disease theories based on spontaneous error, remember that evolution invariably leads to many false conclusions about defective organisms. Don't be deceived by fancy terminology like "hypercholesteremia." Big words often obscure faulty science.

Brenda, a patient of mine, sent me the following message: *Doctors make us afraid of our own bodies. This is precisely what I've been going through almost my entire life, in mortal fear of the enemy: my body.*

In truth, our bodies are our number-one ally, not our worst enemy.

DISPROVEN HEART DISEASE THEORIES

During my undergraduate studies at Brooklyn College, I took a course called "The Physiology of Stress and Disease," which discussed modern medicine's new theories about the effects stress has on the body. Though the ideas were interesting, the course frustrated me since the science was so new; it seemed that they were grappling in the dark.

When I first began studying Chinese medicine, it was like learning a new language. Literally. I had to learn Chinese. Learning Chinese medical theory, it became clear to me that, unlike the patronizing and uninformed view many in the West have of it, Chinese medicine is a complete, advanced medical system. In addition, it is logical. While the terms were foreign, the concepts were universal. Treating patients during my clinical internship, I saw that Chinese medicine worked not only in theory, but in practice as well.

I'm always surprised the public has so much faith in "the latest research," since new discoveries consistently disprove previously held scientific tenets — and they happen at an alarming pace!

> *After her baby was born, Debbie was offered vitamin K and hepatitis B shots for her newborn, which she declined. The doctor tried to convince her that not following hospital protocol would endanger her baby.*
>
> *She asked him, "Doctor, do you read medical journals from ten years ago?"*
>
> *"Of course not!" he responded. "I only trust the latest research."*
>
> *"Well, doctor, in ten years from now, what you are telling me will be ten years old!"*

One of the reasons I chose to study Chinese medicine was because its two thousand years of experience gives it the advantage of being beyond the experimental phase. It became clear to me that modern medicine was just scratching the surface of many long-understood medical concepts.

"SOFT SCIENCE"

For a hundred years, cholesterol and saturated fats have been incriminated as the source of heart disease. Yet there is no scientific evidence to back up the original hypothesis.

In 1988, the US surgeon general's office decided to gather all the evidence to prove the diet-heart hypothesis with finality. Eleven years later, the project was dropped. Word was that the office "did not anticipate the magnitude of the additional expertise and staff resources that would be needed." In eleven years, with the US government's unlimited budget, they were unable to scrape together sufficient evidence to prove a one-hundred-year-old hypothesis.

Bill Harlan, associate director of the Office of Disease Prevention at the NIH (National Institute of Health), commented, "The report was initiated with a preconceived opinion of the conclusions [that cholesterol and saturated fat cause heart disease], but the science behind those opinions was clearly not holding up."[59]

So what's causing heart disease?

One common denominator that has consistently been found in scientific studies is **stress**. The stress hormone cortisol triggers blood-vessel damage and even acute blood clots. Chinese medicine has explained that stress is one of the major causes of heart disease for two millennia.

POPULATIONS UNDER STRESS

According to Dr. Malcolm Kendrick, populations that experience major stress on a national level usually have a high incidence of heart disease. For example, where populations were displaced (i.e., forced out of their homes, separated from family, and generally mistreated), the results were always an increase in heart disease:

- The Australian natives, the Aborigines, began suffering from unusually high rates of heart disease as a result of oppression.
- Sadly, despite being at the cutting edge of medicine and having low average cholesterol levels, Israel has a very high rate of heart disease. I am sure you can imagine why.

---

59   Gary Taubes, "The Soft Science of Dietary Fat," *Science*, 30 Mar 2001: Vol. 291, Issue 5513, pp. 2536–2545.

If you want to reduce heart-disease risk, evidence shows that:

- Eating lots of fruits and vegetables seems to reduce heart-disease incidence.
- Exercise has also been shown to reduce the risk of heart attack, as well as many other diseases. Enjoyable exercise is also an antidote to stress.
- Smoking is a proven risk factor for heart disease.
- Stress: If there are things in your life that are causing a constant state of tension, do something about it. It may save your life.

12

FEVER

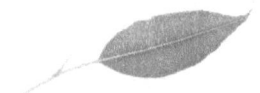

Hanna, *a friend of mine who lives in New York, is decidedly natural-minded. A while back, when Hanna's daughter had a fever, she did not want to give her Tylenol. Hanna's mother, a fan of modern medicine, was very concerned that her daughter was endangering her child. She went as far as calling Hanna's pediatrician (a well-known doctor in Brooklyn) to tattle on her daughter for not giving Tylenol to her granddaughter. She was surprised when the doctor responded, "I'm not supposed to tell you this, but your daughter is doing the right thing."*

What's the big secret this doctor is keeping? If there is reason to believe that giving fever reducers is not good medicine, wouldn't we all like to know about it?

Fevers are one of the main criteria by which people define illness. Some think that the height of a fever is an indication of the severity of the disease. In truth:

- Some mild illnesses, like roseola, can be accompanied by very high fevers.
- Other frightening diseases, like pertussis (whooping cough), are not associated with fever at all.

SEIZURES

One reason that people are afraid of high fevers is because they are associated with seizures. There is a connection, but it is not a *high* fever that causes seizures, but a *rapidly elevating temperature*. These seizures are rarely preventable because the first symptom to alert parents to the severity of the illness is not the fever, but often the seizure itself.

A child with a sustained high fever is not at great risk of having a seizure. Febrile seizures (seizures occurring as the result of rapidly elevated temperature), while frightening to behold, are usually not dangerous and do not necessarily indicate that the child is on the road to a seizure disorder (aka epilepsy). Seizures can occur as a one-time fluke and may not necessarily recur during future illnesses. Seizures are merely a symptom of a disease that may need proper diagnosis; suppressing a fever or a seizure will not treat the underlying problem. Giving seizure medication to a child who has a one-time febrile seizure can set a bad precedent. Give the child a chance to recover from the illness, and presume the child is *not* epileptic unless recurring symptoms indicate otherwise.

SYMPTOMS THAT INDICATE DANGER

While height of temperature is no indication of disease severity, there are some symptoms that signify that a child may be in danger and emergency care is needed. These include difficulty breathing, vomiting, and/or diarrhea to the point of dehydration, abnormal behavior, and confusion.

Beware of symptoms of meningitis, which include a persistent headache, vomiting, fever, and possibly convulsions. Neck stiffness, which is associated with meningitis, does not always occur, and is often present in harmless cases of common cold or flu. The salient symptom is a shrill cry. A high-pitched and eerie cry may also occur after the DTaP vaccination and is a sign of brain inflammation, which is essentially the same thing as meningitis or encephalitis. Mothers are often the best judges about the severity of their children's illnesses. Trust your instincts.

Perhaps the main reason we commonly fear fever is the belief that if not checked with medication, a fever will continue to escalate out of control. In fact, a fever that occurs in response to infection is an important part of our immune response. Our bodies have a built-in mechanism that will not allow a fever to reach 106 degrees Fahrenheit. A fever that lasts many days is a reason to call your pediatrician, pediatric acupuncturist, or homeopath. But keeping hydrated and waiting it out is also fine for experienced moms. For inexperienced moms, a visit from Bubby (Grandma) may be advised.

BAD FEVERS

The only time a fever can rise dangerously is if it was induced by an outside stimulus such as poisoning or hyperthermia (such as sunstroke or sauna overuse). These situations require emergency medical attention. There is also a strange phenomenon that can occur in some children after vaccination, where fevers can rise dangerously high (above 106°F). These fevers may be accompanied by seizures as well. Vaccine-induced seizures often *do* lead to epilepsy, and everything I said above goes out the window when it comes to fevers occurring as vaccine reactions.

Firstly, although febrile seizures do not generally lead to epilepsy, vaccine-induced seizures often *do*. Secondly, in the presence of vaccines, the body's mechanism to prevent escalating temperatures can be severely hampered. Fevers associated with vaccination are not of the natural variety, since the disease is being introduced via an abnormal route (i.e., injection). Therefore, vaccination may override the body's built-in defense mechanisms, in which case a fever may actually skyrocket in an unnatural and dangerous fashion.

GOOD FEVERS

The body produces fevers to help fight infection. When the body temperature rises, immune function is working. Fevers inhibit viral and bacterial growth, and speed up the metabolism. Artificially induced fevers have even shown great promise in the treatment of cancer. In the words of world-renowned oncologist Dr. Josef Issels, "Artificially induced fever has the greatest potential in the treatment of many diseases, including cancer." While a fever often means that a child is ill, it rarely means that the child is in danger.

So should we give our children Tylenol? Fever reducers are palliative at best, as they may relieve some discomfort. However, in many cases they are a poor choice, as they actually *suppress* immune function and can prevent the body from recovering from the illness, and prolong the recovery time.

13

STREP
THROAT

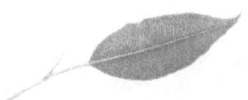

Anumber of years ago, I wrote an article for a magazine on the subject of Chinese medicine and acupuncture. I mentioned that Chinese medicine can "treat conditions ranging from strep throat to indigestion to insomnia."

The following week, a doctor wrote an irate letter in response to my article. The physician felt that it was irresponsible to suggest alternative treatments for strep throat, mentioning the potential danger of untreated strep developing into rheumatic fever. While this has been accepted as a hard fact, many are unaware that the connection between strep throat and rheumatic fever is an unproven theory.

Setting rheumatic fever aside for the moment, this doctor believed that employing options other than antibiotics leaves the condition "untreated."

I beg to differ. There are plenty of alternatives to antibiotics that work. They are often much more effective than antibiotics in the long run. In defense of the "rebels" who seek assistance from holistic health practitioners, most of them do so because they are suffering from chronically recurring infection. Most of them have taken antibiotics many times. Some have even been prescribed a continuous low dose of antibiotics.

And yet the infection keeps returning! These children (or adults) are often not *catching* strep; the disease lies dormant in their body. In chronic cases, the bacteria "come back to life" and strike again. Even the biggest fans of modern medicine seek alternatives when tonsillectomy (surgical removal of the tonsils) becomes the only remaining option...

While antibiotics certainly have their place and may on occasion be lifesaving, repeated courses often become ineffective or even harmful. Firstly, they create drug-resistant bacteria. What used to be a theoretical concern has now become a reality: The CDC (Centers for Disease Control) is constantly reporting new strains of super-bacteria that are impervious to antibiotics. Aside from strep throat, antibiotics are overprescribed for a myriad of sometimes only *potential* conditions.

Antibiotics also kill the beneficial gut flora (good bacteria), which is responsible for healthy digestion. Probiotics can balance out this effect somewhat. Live yogurt can also be given at a dose of one teaspoon three times a day during the course of antibiotics and for three days after completion. This amount of yogurt is all that is needed to introduce healthy bacteria. Larger quantities of yogurt can be unhealthy for many children.

Why do illnesses become chronic in some people?

Western medicine understands conditions like tonsillitis to be the result of a bacterial or viral infection. But if microorganisms were the only factor involved, there would be a far greater incidence of strep throat, being that strep has been found living in the tonsils of many well individuals! The real question is: Why do some people get sick from the bacteria living in their bodies, while others remain completely healthy in the presence of the very same microorganisms?

The obvious answer is that it depends a lot more on the state of the body than the presence of microorganisms. For example, of the very large number of people who have been exposed to the Epstein-Barr virus (as indicated by antibodies in the bloodstream), only a small percentage suffer from debilitating illness (mononucleosis).

It is not the virus that causes exhaustion, but exhaustion that allows the virus to take hold. Diet and emotions also influence the body's internal environment and can play an important role in illness. Poor eating habits, especially junk food, can weaken a person and may even feed infection.

Regarding emotions, frustration or anger can be contributing factors to chronic tonsillitis. Tonsillitis is not commonly seen in infants under two years old, but it often appears between the ages of two and three. Chinese medicine explains that the reason for this phenomenon is that at this age, children experience a lot of frustration (think terrible twos); they are struggling to communicate, and attempting to accomplish a lot of things but are often unsuccessful. At the age of six or seven, there may be another upsurge of tonsillitis, since this is an age when a child becomes more emotionally self-aware.

While the approach of modern medicine is to vanquish the pathogen (i.e., kill the bacteria), traditional medicine looks *first and foremost* at the body's environment. While there are herbs that can kill microorganisms, the treatment almost always takes into account remedies to strengthen the body so that it is capable of eliminating the pathogen and protecting itself from future infection.

While antibiotics may kill the bad guys (though their effects are weaker and weaker with each passing day), to treat and prevent illness, it is often not enough just to kill the bad guys; we must strengthen the good guy too. In modern medicine, the good guy is the pharmaceutical drug, while in traditional medicine the good guy is you.

Keep in mind that even those without chronic recurrence who choose natural treatments for strep are not actually being irresponsible. In fact, those who have not taken repeated courses of antibiotics generally respond much faster when administered natural holistic remedies.

How do I know if it's really strep throat?

A couple of months ago, Leah brought her three-year-old daughter, Shana, to see me. She told me, "She has chronic strep throat. She's been on and off antibiotics for virtually all her life and I'd like to get rid of it once and for all."

I asked Leah for more details, and she told me that every time Shana came down with a cold, she would take a strep culture, and it would come out positive, so she was taking antibiotics every few weeks.

"Does she complain of throat pain?" I asked her.

"Not usually," Leah responded.

"Do her tonsils appear red, inflamed, spotty, or filled with pus?"

"I don't know, we never really checked."

"Well, let's have a look right now."

I inspected Shana's tonsils and they looked normal. I told her that a positive strep test does not necessarily indicate a genuine strep infection, especially in the absence of the above symptoms.

If I would culture one hundred symptomless people right now, some of them would probably test positive for strep throat. Many people are carrying strep bacteria without it making them sick. And it may never cause any symptoms.

Although Shana was testing positive for strep, she did not have any symptoms associated with strep-throat infection. Her symptoms were probably caused by a virus, and the strep found was not related to her current state. I told Leah that I suspected that Shana was not suffering from chronic strep throat at all — just chronic overdiagnosis of strep, and lots of unnecessary antibiotics.

I treated Shana and told Leah that once the cold passed, as long as no symptoms of tonsillitis developed (very sore throat, painful swallowing, swollen red tonsils with discharge or white patches...), there was no need to even get a culture. I also suggested some minor dietary changes to boost Shana's immune function and prevent her from catching even non-strep infections. (She switched from sweet breakfast cereals to fresh fruit smoothies.)

A few months later, I got a call from Leah. "How's your daughter?" I inquired. She was fine; she hadn't experienced another strep "alarm" since her last appointment. She just wanted to bring in her son who was under the weather. I was happy that my instincts were correct and the story ended well. (Leah told me that now Shana will not go a day without her fresh fruit smoothies. Seems like the start of a fun and healthy family tradition.)

While they can be effective in individual cases of bacterial infection, antibiotics are often prescribed too hastily and broadly, with little recognition of their potential harm. I wish it were as simple as they make it seem: "Bad bacteria invade and make us ill. Antibiotics kill the disease and restore us to good health."

Antibiotics don't just kill bad bacteria; they kill all nonresistant strains, including healthy bacteria. Our first line of immune defense is in the gut, in the form of stomach acids and good bacteria. Wiping out our good gut flora can actually make us more prone to infection since the good bacteria seem to keep the bad bacteria in check.

The long-term effects of antibiotics are often even worse than the short term.

Antibiotics are one of the major causes of obesity today. Did you know that antibiotics are given to farm animals not just to kill infection, but to fatten them up?

Infections rarely erupt spontaneously. They are usually the result of an unhealthy bodily environment. For example, when scientists tested corn-fed cows, their guts were found to be riddled with unhealthy E. coli bacteria. When these cows were fed grass for a few weeks, the E. coli vanished! A positive change in diet allowed the cows to restore proper gut bacteria. This is something antibiotics cannot do.

Sadly, over the years I have seen many people who are suffering from chronic illness because of antibiotic overuse. The worst cases are usually those who took antibiotics the longest. Many people come to me to fix the damage that was done after years of health-debilitating treatments. They tell me heart-wrenching stories of how their health deteriorated further with each intervention. After years like this, they begin to pursue natural alternatives.

A word of advice: Try natural treatments before pursuing extreme interventions that can sometimes lead to years of endless and ever-escalating treatments. It is much easier to cure a patient with natural medicine when they do not have a lifelong history of pharmaceutical treatment. This is one of the reasons that little children are so much more responsive — their systems are much less encumbered. These days, more and more conventional doctors are recommending natural or nutritional treatments. They see the need to step out of the antibiotic box now that their effectiveness is declining so rapidly. Few doctors seem to be aware that there are other problems with antibiotics besides decreasing effectiveness. Their role in causing chronic disease needs more attention.

See the home-remedies section for more on prevention and treatment of acute sore throat.

14

SINUS
INFECTIONS

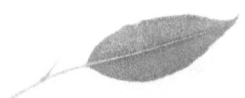

There are numerous conditions that are labeled "infections" that may not be due to microorganisms at all. These include: sinus infections, ear infections, mastitis, pneumonia, and even many cases of bronchitis. What all these conditions have in common is an accumulation of fluids or mucus. This mucus then becomes a breeding ground for bacteria. Often, the mucus was there first, and the organisms make themselves a home in this ready medium secondarily. If you can clear out the mucus or fluid buildup, the infection will automatically be flushed out in the process.

Many people suffer from recurring sinus infections. Why do they recur, even after antibiotic treatment?

Antibiotics only kill bacteria (unless the bacteria are resistant); they do not cleanse the body of the pathogenic environment. On the contrary, in my experience antibiotics not only tend to weaken our body's immune response, but can actually promote mucus production. Additionally, they decimate the digestive systems of many susceptible individuals, especially babies and children.

While antibiotics may cause a sinus infection to die down, thereby eliminating inflammation and pain, for many people this relief is only temporary. As long as the congestion remains, it is only a matter of time before the bacteria set up residence again.

There are certain factors that make some individuals more susceptible than others. One thing I have observed is that some kids on stimulants like Ritalin or Concerta can get sinus infections often. It is, in fact, a known adverse reaction that may be somewhat more common than the package insert suggests.

There are several ways to eliminate chronic sinus infections so that they do not recur:

1. **Eliminate foods that promote mucus**. Trigger foods may include: dairy, peanut butter, bananas, orange juice, white sugar, and wheat. Mucus-producing foods vary from one individual to another, but these foods nearly always cause trouble. I frequently come across individuals with chronic sinus trouble who are dairy addicts. Many of my patients have reported that after eliminating dairy, their health improved dramatically.

   In any adult or child with a mucus condition, try removing dairy from your diet. If you are not congested with phlegm and do not have lactose or casein intolerance, dairy may not hurt you as much — some people can handle it better than others. Still, this step alone often solves mucus and sinus problems. Read further to learn about other good sources of calcium.

2. **Sinus wash**. There are various ways to do this. By forcefully squirting a saline solution (i.e., salty water) up your nose, you can wash the mucus right out of your sinuses. Some people have great success with this method.

   Use warm filtered water and a bit of salt. You can use a neti pot, a nasal dropper, or a water bottle with a narrow spout. Introduce the water into one nostril with strong pressure while tilting your head forward and away from that nostril. If you do it right, the water will exit from the other nostril or the mouth. This can be a jarring experience at first, but it gets easier. For chronic sinus trouble, repeat this process daily or as often as possible for several weeks or months.

3. **Citrus Seed Extract,** which can be used as a nasal spray, has a good reputation as a broad spectrum, yet gentle, antimicrobial.

4. **Acupuncture.** Many of my patients, even or especially those who do not follow the preceding advice, experience immediate relief in their sinus infections after receiving acupuncture. If you're afraid of needles, go back to 1 through 3.

NOTE ABOUT NEEDLES

I get the following question very often: "Does acupuncture hurt?"

The simple answer is, "It depends." Those who are sensitive (like redheads?) may feel the needle insertion more distinctly than those who are less sensitive or have a higher pain threshold.

I once heard a story about some college students who tried acupuncture at a student clinic that used particularly fine needles. They reported back to another acupuncturist excitedly that they "felt nothing!" Well, the acupuncturist said, "If you felt nothing, then the treatment probably did nothing, because when acupuncture works, you feel it."

Though the feeling that acupuncture elicits is not usually painful, sometimes (fleetingly) acupuncture can hurt a little. If that scares you, take Tylenol. (Seriously. When mothers bring in their sick babies to me and have given them fever reducers, the babies rarely feel the acupuncture. I'm not entirely sure that this is a good thing, but it makes everybody much happier.)

I was administering a particularly unique and painful treatment (on the palms and soles!) upon a very motivated patient, and continuously apologized to her about the pain (most other points on the body don't hurt at all, and I rarely choose these points without clear necessity and tremendous motivation from my patient). She said, "I want the treatment because I hope it will help me, why should a little pain scare me?"

Here's the thing: while the purpose of acupuncture is not to cause pain, the goal of acupuncture is not specifically to be painless. For a pain-free existence, you can sit on your couch, which wouldn't hurt at all (unless you sit too long, which can ache a little)! The purpose of acupuncture is to produce results and improve health. I find that with that end goal in mind, even a bit of transient pain (we are talking seconds) may be worthwhile. Of course, it is a matter of preference.

Just to be fair, I acknowledge that needles are scary with or without pain. In fact, most of my patients are not at all afraid of a painful massage, even if it's much more painful than acupuncture. There is just something about needles that people find…unfriendly. And I can't blame them. Keep in mind, a graduate-school classmate of mine once said, "I used to go for acupressure (massage of acupuncture points), but I had to quit because it was just too painful." Instead, she opted for acupuncture — because it hurt less.

So although acupuncture is admittedly a little frightening, it is almost always less painful than a massage, and even if there is pain, it usually only lasts for a few seconds.

15

COUGH

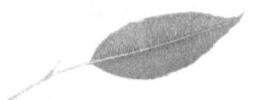

Patients often visit my clinic complaining of a "cold" that they can't seem to get rid of. By the time they come to see me, however, it is usually weeks after they contracted the infection. The one or two symptoms that remain are really the baggage left behind by a virus that has already passed through. In reality, the cold itself is gone; it is stubborn mucus that remains. This mucus is commonly found in the form of a lingering cough.

> *Evelyn brought her three-year-old daughter, Molly, to me to treat her cough. Aside from giving her acupuncture and herbs, I told Evelyn that Molly should abstain from dairy until her lungs were completely clear.*
>
> *During the next visit, Molly was still coughing. Upon inquiry, Evelyn revealed that she had continued providing dairy. "How can I take all dairy out of her diet?" she questioned. "She won't get enough calcium!" I responded that when a child's breathing is compromised, we do not look at long-term nutrition, only the immediate effect of the foods consumed.*

The poor quality of cow's milk products available today makes them an unhealthful choice for many people. Luckily, there are some good sources of calcium besides dairy. I have listed the following foods in descending order that, gram for gram, supply more calcium than dairy. This list is by no means exhaustive (and numbers have been rounded).

Milk contains about 119 mg of calcium per 100-gram serving. The figures below indicate how many times more calcium than milk each of the following foods contain per serving.

	Number of times more calcium than milk	*Mg of calcium per 100-gram (3-oz.) serving*
Kelp	9	1100
Sesame seeds	9	1110
Sardines	3.7	452
Almonds	2	244
Amaranth	2	244
Parsley	1.7	208
Sunflower seeds	1.5	183
Chickpeas	1.25	152
Quinoa	1.2	147
Black beans	1.13	138
Pistachios	1.1	134
Dried figs	1.06	130

Note: Hard cheese contains about 5.7 times more calcium than milk, and is sometimes tolerated by people who cannot digest milk. (This is probably because the ratio of the allergenic proteins like lactose and casein are higher in milk, whereas in many cheeses the fat content is higher, and allergy-triggering proteins are lower.) Of course, if all dairy is a problem, there is no need to worry about malnutrition because, as you can see, there are plenty of nondairy foods that contain large amounts of calcium.

Dairy produces mucus. When a child is wheezing, mucus is clogging their breathing passages. The benefits of calcium are completely outweighed by the dangerous increase of mucus that dairy produces. For chronic coughs or runny nose or asthma, avoid dairy "chronically" and replace the calcium with another source. Children with coughs should also avoid other phlegm-producing foods such as bananas, peanut butter, white flour, and white sugar.

MY DAUGHTER'S CROUPY COUGH

A while back, our fifteen-month-old developed a frightening dry cough in the middle of the night. I took her out of bed and gave her acupuncture. I usually see an immediate improvement after acupuncture, but this cough was stubborn. For the next hour, I gave her warm water with honey, and an acupressure massage. I then put her back to bed. By the next morning, her cough was 90 percent better.

Not all coughs are the same. Some are wet and some are dry. Honey would have made a wet cough worse, but for a dry cough, it was beneficial. Pear juice is also particularly helpful for lubricating a dry cough; it is used medicinally in Chinese medicine for this condition. Dry coughs are more common in dry desert climates.

Sandra came to me for treatment for a lingering dry cough. She asked me if she should abstain from dairy. I suggested that after the treatment she should try avoiding dairy and report back to me. She called me a few days later and told me that the cough was almost gone. However, when she had some dairy, the cough started to get worse again.

Even though dairy is moistening, it usually produces moisture in the form of unhealthy phlegm, so it is not good for any kind of cough.

PREGNANCY COUGHS

I received a call from Aliza, who was at the end of her ninth month of pregnancy. She had caught a bad cold that was lingering stubbornly (a common occurrence during pregnancy) and had left her with clogged sinuses and lungs. She had taken antibiotics, but they had not helped at all. She was very nervous to go into labor while her breathing was still compromised.

Based on her symptoms, I wrote a very simple herbal formula, which would be safe to use during pregnancy. I told her to start taking it as soon as possible. A few days later, her mother called to tell me that Aliza had taken the herbs for about a day and a half, and then went into labor able to breathe easily once again. She gave birth to a healthy baby boy.

Often, women experience lingering congestion during pregnancy. When breathing is affected, it can be very distressing. Doctors are rightfully hesitant to prescribe drugs, since many pharmaceuticals can be unsafe during pregnancy. There are many herbs that are also forbidden for pregnancy, but luckily there are plenty that are safe. An experienced herbalist can carefully choose herbs that will keep both mother and baby safe.

So keep in mind that every cough is different and must be treated individually. Try to differentiate between whether it is dry or moist, and use home remedies accordingly. One of the biggest errors I see in modern medicine when it comes to coughs is the lack of differentiation on this factor, i.e., they always aim to dry out the mucus, without realizing that sometimes the lungs are already dry, and further drying will create a mucus that is the consistency of hardening glue. Not a good thing.

GAUGING A DRY OR WET COUGH BY THIRST LEVEL:

- Feeling thirsty — means it's a dry cough. It will usually be accompanied by a thick mucus that is difficult to expectorate (cough up). Try moistening it with honey or pear juice.
- Not thirsty — Sometimes accompanied by nausea, this would be labeled a "damp" cough in Chinese medicine, in which case drying herbs or medications are appropriate.

COLORS

In modern medicine, there is a notion — whether in sinus/nasal mucus or the sputum that is coughed up from the chest — that yellow or green color means infection, while clear mucus means you're "in the clear." This is not entirely accurate. Even bloody or brown mucus may not be accompanied by bacterial infection, though sometimes it is.

I suspect that the reason for this differentiation is simply because there is no consistent treatment for mucus in modern medicine unless it becomes infected, in which case antibiotics are prescribed.

Luckily, coughs, especially when they become chronic, can be treated with herbal medicine whether there is a bacterial infection or not. The presence of bacteria is in no way the determining factor to necessitate treatment.

So the color of the mucus does not mean there's an emergency, but there are some factors that should send you to your healthcare provider, even if only one of these symptoms is present:

- Cough has become chronic — lasting more than one week or ten days, and not showing any signs of improvement.
- There is some difficulty or discomfort with breathing.
- Chest pain or tightness associated with coughing.
- Worsening of symptoms over a one-week period or more.
- Fever associated with the cough, especially with a worsening of symptoms.

In the absence of all of the above symptoms, colored mucus is no reason to be concerned. But it does mean something. In Chinese medicine, the color of the mucus indicates the temperature of the condition. So that:

- Yellow or green mucus means a *hot* condition, to be treated with cooling herbs;
- White or clear mucus means a *cold* condition, where the body needs a warming treatment.

Usually, the color of the mucus will be accompanied by more subjective symptoms of hot and cold as well. The cold person will feel cold, even if they have a high temperature. They will be huddling under their blankets and shivering even if it's warm outside (in extreme cases), while the person with a hot type of condition will feel hot, sweaty, thirsty, and will be throwing off their blankets, with or without a high fever.

I like to treat coughs with acupuncture. It works especially well for acute (newer) cases. If acupuncture is not enough, herbs usually do the job, but a correct diagnosis is crucial, as there is no one remedy that suits all coughs. If someone with a dry cough would take a drying remedy, the cough would get worse. If someone with a hot constitution took a warming herb (think cinnamon, ginger, or cayenne pepper) it would be very bad for them.

Here's a silly story that once happened to me when I wasn't paying attention. I was suffering from a sore throat, so my husband (who has a colder constitution) suggested I take lots of black pepper. Well, I have a warmer constitution, and warming herbs are *not* good for me. But, like I said, I wasn't paying attention, so I tried a whole lot of black pepper without really contemplating what the consequences would be, and what do you know? The sore throat got much worse really fast.

While herbal home remedies can sometimes be really effective and really great, if they are a mismatch with the person's constitution, they will be of no benefit and may even be (mildly) harmful. With a better understanding of what the symptoms tell us about the nature of the illness, we can choose home remedies that suit each individual's constitution with greater success.

16

ANTIBIOTICS

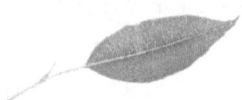

As more and more strains of bacteria are becoming resistant to antibiotics, the CDC (Centers for Disease Control and Prevention) admits that antibiotics are not a long-term solution, being that they are the cause of resistance. The CDC anticipates that in the next few decades, antibiotics will be powerless in fighting many (if not most) forms of bacterial infection. As of now, there are no new antibiotics on the horizon. We are already beginning to pay for their overuse.[60]

The CDC further warns that indiscriminate overuse of antibiotics has caused many strains of bacteria to become resistant, and it is currently working to tamp down unnecessary use of antibiotics. It may come as no surprise that most deaths caused by antibiotic resistant infections occur in hospitals and nursing homes, according to the CDC.[61] What is left unsaid is that ironically, hospitals are breeding grounds for "super-bugs," making them hazardous places for sick people or pregnant women to enter!

Antibiotic resistance is a concept that is misunderstood by many

---

60   "Antibiotic / Antimicrobial Resistance," CDC, April 6, 2017. https://www.cdc.gov/drugresistance/about.html.

61   Ibid.

people, including some doctors: It is not the *person* who develops the resistance, but the *bacteria*. Bacteria are very resilient little creatures. When they are exposed to antibiotics, the ones that survive learn how to defend themselves from these drugs in the future. This is why over time, the same antibiotics have become less and less effective in killing bacteria that they once easily annihilated.

ACCORDING TO THE CDC

The use of antibiotics is the single most important factor leading to antibiotic resistance around the world. Simply using antibiotics creates resistance. These drugs should only be used to manage infections.

Antibiotics are among the most commonly prescribed drugs used in human medicine and can be lifesaving drugs. However, up to 50 percent of the time, antibiotics are not optimally prescribed, often done so when not needed, with incorrect dosing or duration.

Penicillin, the first commercialized antibiotic, was discovered in 1928 by Alexander Fleming. While it wasn't distributed among the general public until 1945, it was widely used in World War II for surgical and wound infections among the Allied Forces. It was hailed as a "miracle drug," and a future free of infectious diseases was considered. When Fleming won the Nobel Prize for his discovery, he warned of bacteria becoming resistant to penicillin in his acceptance speech.

In fact, according to this same CDC report, staphylococcus was already showing resistance to penicillin in 1940, three years *before* it was introduced to the general public![62]

---

62   Ibid.

The overuse of antibiotics gives many bacteria the opportunity to adapt, making many forms of antibiotics increasingly ineffective. Antibiotic overuse does not only mean individuals overdosing, but the massive-scale use of these drugs on billions of people and farm animals worldwide. This includes internal as well as external use. Even antibiotic soaps are contributing to drug resistance.

Antibiotic overuse is often called one of the world's greatest health threats. Still, there is really no reason to be afraid. Let us go back to the time when modern medicine was in its infancy. One of its most famous tenets is the **germ theory**, which takes us to the very heart of modern medicine. Though some argue that it was plagiarized, history gives credit to Louis Pasteur, who claimed that microorganisms are solely responsible for disease. The generally accepted understanding is that all people are born equally susceptible to infection if exposed to microorganisms, that microorganisms invade indiscriminately from the environment, and that the way to cure the infection is to kill the microorganisms. Sickness, according to the germ theory, means invasion of germs or disease.

This line of reasoning has created the treatment principles for all areas of modern medicine, even when infection is not involved. For example:

- The goal of cancer treatment is to attack and kill the cancer.
- If someone suffers from Crohn's disease and is experiencing bowel inflammation, a perfectly acceptable course of action is to remove a portion of the bowel (resection).[63]

The fact that these treatments can be devastating to overall health does not seem to act as much of a deterrent, as long as the goal of fighting or removing the disease is met. The germ theory is a vast over-simplification of reality, as you will soon see.

What were the other guys saying?

In the mid-1800s Professor Pierre Jacque Antoine Bechamp, a con-temporary of Pasteur, presented the **cellular theory**. He asserted that

---

63 I have treated many patients who suffered terribly from scar tissue and intestinal blockage after this procedure.

disease only arises after the health of the (human) host has deteriorated. Disease is created by unhealthy conditions, and germs (bacteria, viruses, fungi, or parasites) will only cause illness when health is lacking. He postulated that the way to prevent disease is to create health.

While the germ theory won out in the short-term, and still enjoys world renown, Pasteur's simplistic hypothesis was disproved many times over.

- In the 1920s, when Dr. Royal R. Rife of San Diego, California, invented a powerful microscope, he discovered that bacteria could change from beneficial to harmful depending on the medium in which they were placed.
- Scientists have found that harmless bacteria can become disease-causing and vice versa. According to an article in Scientific American:

> Bacteria are all around — and inside — us. Some are harmless, some are beneficial, and some, of course, cause disease. Others, such as the common bacterium Streptococcus pneumoniae, defy categorization. They are turncoats, with the ability to suddenly switch from good to bad. Usually the microbe dwells harmlessly in people's nasal passages. Every so often, however, when S. pneumoniae senses danger, it disperses to other areas of the body in a bid to save itself, making us sick.[64]

  Although Scientific American's explanation for why this is remains murky, Bechamp's long-unrecognized hypothesis perfectly explains why this happens.
- Around a century ago at the Mayo Clinic, world-renowned dentist Dr. Weston Price discovered that deadly anaerobic bacteria can spawn in dead teeth that are anchored into the mouth via

64   Robyn Braun, "When Harmless Bacteria Go Bad," *Scientific American*, December 1, 2013.

root canals. Unbelievably, after removing root-canal teeth from chronically ill patients, he implanted them under the skin of rabbits. The rabbits then developed the same disease the person had, including heart attack, cancer, and neurological disease!

> The American Dental Association (ADA) denies his findings and claims that they have proven root canals to be safe; however, no published data from the ADA is available to confirm this statement.[65]

This terribly complicates our understanding of the effects bad bacteria can have on overall health, but is mentioned here specifically to explain how a bad environment (i.e., a dead tooth left in the mouth) can spawn disease-causing microorganisms.

The germ theory puts no obligation on the individual to preserve his health. According to the theory, disease is an external force that has no relation to the choices you make, as opposed to being an inevitable consequence of an unhealthful lifestyle. People who believed this theory erroneously thought that should disease spontaneously erupt, the individual would be powerless against it. Only their doctor would be able to help with "a pill for every ill." Modern medicine has come around quite a bit, and most doctors today understand the importance of diet and lifestyle in promoting health (as Bechamp said over 150 years ago and Chinese medicine has been saying for thousands of years).

I have my own hypothesis that I'd like to share: I suggest that in many cases, modern medicine has reality perfectly reversed. In modern medicine, diseases that are caused by nature are blamed on the body, and diseases that are rooted in the body are blamed on nature. For example:

- Not everyone who is exposed to a cold or flu virus will become ill. It will depend greatly on overall health. Though illness here may require some external exposure, the internal bodily

---

65   Hal Huggins, DDS, MS, *Root Canal Dangers*, Weston A. Price Foundation, June 25, 2010.

environment is of utmost importance and will determine individual susceptibility.

- Measles, mumps, rubella, and chicken pox are blamed on viruses and are considered to be externally contracted diseases. However, in homeopathic medicine and in Chinese medicine, these diseases are considered *an intrinsic part of pediatric development*! They are said to expel toxins that babies pick up in the womb ("fetal toxins"), and act as gateways toward *improving* health. Once again, this is an interplay between external exposure and the internal environment.

- Viruses are very poorly understood entities; they are strands of RNA, basically codes — not life forms at all. So all they can really do to their host is *relay information*! Some viruses are intrinsic to humans, and are rarely or never found in animals, which strongly suggests that these diseases are not simply externally contracted infectious agents, but something far more complex.

On the other hand:

- Cancer is often blamed on human defects, like genetics, when in fact most cancers are caused by exposure to toxic carcinogens. Cancer is truly an externally caused disease. Now I am going to unfairly include an example of how a virus can be a cause of cancer. But in this particular case, the virus was not intrinsic to humans; it was unnaturally introduced between 1955 and 1961 when it contaminated polio vaccines that were incubated in rhesus monkey cell cultures. The SV-40 (the 40th simian virus discovered) was introduced into millions of people through polio vaccination, and is a major carcinogen, with mesotheliomas being the most common form of cancer triggered.[66]

---

66   Fisher SG, Weber L, Carbone M., "Cancer risk associated with simian virus 40 contaminated polio vaccine," *Anticancer Res.* 1999 May–Jun;19(3B):2173-80. https://www.ncbi.nlm.nih.gov/pubmed/10472327.

These data suggest that there may be an increased incidence of certain cancers among the **ninety-eight million persons exposed** to contaminated polio vaccine in the US [emphasis added].[67]

The SV-40 virus was harmless to monkeys and would have been impossible to spread to other species without incubating and then injecting monkey tissue into humans. I suspect that this RNA is simply a normal strand of information in monkey kidneys and contains instructions that are harmless to rhesus monkeys, and is harmful to us simply because it is out of place in the human body.

Few back then grasped that these vaccines might also be a huge, inadvertent, uncontrolled experiment in interspecies viral transmission.[68] [69]

(HIV is yet another virus that was transferred from monkeys [SIV — Simian Immunodeficiency Virus] to humans, mainly through vaccination, as monkey kidneys were used as an incubation medium for polio vaccines. In monkeys, this virus did not cause disease. It was only when this RNA was unwittingly transferred to humans that a new disease was created.)

- Diseases like multiple sclerosis, Parkinson's disease, Alzheimer's, and many others are considered to be caused largely by genetic defects. In reality, these diseases are caused by exposure to heavy metals like aluminum, mercury, and possibly lead and others, exposure to excitotoxins like MSG and aspartame, and other environmental and external triggers.

---

67   Ibid.

68   Tom Curtis, "Monkeys, viruses, and vaccines," *The Lancet*, Volume 364 , Issue 9432 , 407–408.

69   See also: Debbie Bookchin and Jim Schumacher, *The Virus and the Vaccine: The True Story of a Cancer-Causing Monkey Virus, Contaminated Polio Vaccine, and the Millions of Americans Exposed.*

Holistic medicine is not simply an alternative to antibiotics. It follows an entirely different line of reasoning and understands that it is the body, not the germ, that will predict illness and health.

17

STAYING HEALTHY
WITHOUT MEDICINE

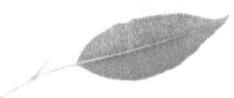

Although I am trained in prescribing Chinese herbal medicine and I love Chinese herbs, since I don't live near a Chinatown, it's not always easy to access herbs, especially for daily use and minor ailments. For that reason (and based on the recommendation of a homeopathic doctor I was working with at the time), I bought a one-hundred-remedies homeopathic kit, which is much easier to store at home in a tiny box than hundreds of Chinese herbs!

I'm not an expert in homeopathy, but I own a few books on the subject. One nice book that I have is called *Homeopathic Medicine at Home*, by Maesimund B. Panos, MD, and Jane Heimlich. It is an excellent choice for parents who are interested in using homeopathic home remedies for minor ailments.

There is one paragraph in the (otherwise excellent) book where the authors got it so wrong that if it wasn't so sad it would be funny:

> Judging by the ill-fated swine flu program that began in February of 1976, characterized by bureaucratic confusion and serious side effects, including fatalities, it seems unlikely that the government will attempt another massive campaign to inoculate the public against flu.[70]

Well, history can be rather myopic, and it seems that the 1976 disaster has been utterly forgotten and the effort to vaccinate every sentient being with flu has been reignited with a vengeance.

The flu vaccine carries a rather high risk of causing "flu-like symptoms" (i.e., the flu), and many people have told me that after suffering in bed for a week after their annual flu shot, they decided to opt out of further flu vaccines. The chance of the flu shot actually preventing the flu is rather low as well since the shot may not even match that year's new "recombinant" virus strains. With reports of paralysis, Guillain-Barré syndrome (rapid-onset muscle weakness caused by the immune system damaging the peripheral nervous system), and even death (some of these cases reported to me personally) after flu vaccines, one may wonder if there is a safer way to prevent flu.

> *A relative of mine was filling out a flu-vaccine exemption form for work. On the form, one of the choices listed as reason for opting out of the shot was "A history of Guillain-Barré syndrome." The main if not only cause of Guillain-Barré syndrome is the flu vaccine. It is a condition that is far worse than the flu.*

Influenza is just one disease. Whether the flu is harmless or deadly is subject to continuous debate. However, using health-promoting

---

70   Maesimund B. Panos, MD, and Jane Heimlich, *Homeopathic Medicine at Home*, p. 109.

methods to prevent *all* diseases will invariably protect us from being hurt by the flu as well, to the best of our abilities.

Rather than simply focusing on fighting individual pathogens, which will not make us healthier, we'd best use methods that improve overall health. Once we understand the definition of genuine health, it becomes obvious that preventing or fighting disease with disease-causing agents defies common sense.

Everyone wants to be healthy; most people just don't quite know how to attain health. Some drugs are effective, but what do they accomplish in the long run? Healthy people don't need prescription (or nonprescription) drugs. They don't need pills, injections, or inhalers. The way to prevent and treat disease is to restore health. Since drugs often make people less healthy, they are certainly not capable of eradicating disease. With the overuse of pharmaceuticals, what often happens is that in the process of suppressing one disease, another disease is triggered.

"LET FOOD BE THY MEDICINE AND MEDICINE BE THY FOOD"

For thousands of years, it was common knowledge and common sense that what you eat has the greatest influence on your health. If tiny pills can influence bodily processes, isn't it obvious that what we eat becomes the building blocks for our entire body? Healthy eating habits are not a magic pill, they are our lifeline. People who eat right for their bodies have been able to cure themselves of all types of diseases. Diet makes a difference for nearly all illnesses. There are certain foods that are universally unhealthy, so I will address some of them here.

Foods to Avoid

White sugar has been shown repeatedly to suppress immune function and promote the growth of unhealthy cells, such as bad bacteria, fungi, and even cancer. However, the claim that sugar is even worse than artificial sweeteners is baseless. If you have a choice between artificial or real sugar, throw them both in the garbage. Just kidding. There is no doubt that real sugar is the lesser of two evils. Anyone who says otherwise has not done their homework. Yet sugar intake should be kept to a minimum. Safer alternatives to white sugar include honey, stevia, barley malt, demerara sugar, molasses, and date syrup (a Middle Eastern specialty). Each of these has its advantages and disadvantages.

TIPS TO TEMPER A SWEET TOOTH

- **Stop sweetening savory dishes!** Ever tried meatballs in tomato sauce that did not have loads of sugar added? Ever went a week eating salad dressings that were not sweetened? Ever tried a plain yogurt, or sugarless mayonnaise? We are so used to finding sugar in savory dishes that we don't even know what food would taste like without it. Like the rest of the world, I spent most of my life adding sugar to any food that would allow it, thinking that it would not be edible otherwise. ("The tomato sauce would just be too sour without it!")
  Then I read the following in one of my favorite cookbooks about making things from scratch (*Make the Bread, Buy the Butter* by Jennifer Reese): "Many major producers [of marinara sauce...] add sugar to their marinara and it tastes unwholesome and overly sweet. Plus, the routine sugaring of savory food is annoying." Well, I did not want to be accused of being an annoying chef, so I stopped adding sugar to my savory dishes then and there. Since then, I have acquired a new appreciation for savory dishes without sugar. They actually taste much better than their sugar-bearing counterparts. Some foods are simply weird with added sugar. Why add sugar to pesto? And mayonnaise?
- **Add fat.** Ever noticed that as the fat content goes down, the sugar content goes up? The best example I can think of is overly sweet fat-free yogurt, but there are many. Don't be afraid to add olive oil, butter, or high-quality

cheeses to your dishes. Well-marbled (high-fat) meats were once considered a delicacy. Now they are (falsely) labeled a health hazard. People who eat enough fat crave sugar less, their blood sugar is stabilized, and saturated fat in particular can reverse type 2 diabetes.

Hydrogenated Trans Fats, such as margarine and shortening, replace natural saturated fats in bodily cell structures and promote abnormal cellular activity. They have been implicated in cancer, heart disease, and infertility, among other things. Hydrogenated fats may cause many other chronic illnesses, and should be avoided like the plague.

Preservatives, such as sulfites and sodium benzoate, are used to give foods a longer shelf life. They are chemicals that arrest development of life inside the package...and inside your body.

The use of **artificial sweeteners,** such as sucralose (Splenda), saccharin (Sweet'n Low), and aspartame (Equal) is difficult to justify. If there is even a possibility that they might be carcinogenic, why take the risk? They are certainly not health-promoting, and they don't even taste very good. They may however, be addictive to some people since, according to neurosurgeon Russell Blaylock, MD, many artificial sweeteners are "excitoxins," which means they excite neurons to death and cause neurological diseases such as Alzheimer's and Parkinson's disease.[71]

Even moderate amounts of fake sugar are dangerous. With mounting evidence against these sweeteners, the fact that they've been FDA approved should not act as reassurance of their safety. Avoiding sugar should not mean replacing it with synthetic chemicals. Eat something you love that's not sweet instead.

Dairy, homogenized, pasteurized, antibioticized, hormonized cow's milk is one of the major causes of illness today. Many people's health improves when they go *off* of cow's milk products. On the other hand,

---

71   Russell Blaylock, MD, *Excitotoxins: The Taste That Kills,* 1994.

dairy is not intrinsically bad. The problem is that modern-day dairy production has ruined something that was originally great. Milk from healthy, free-range, grass-fed cows contains important nutrients that are nonexistent in the battery-farmed, corn-fed cow's milk we find on supermarket shelves today.

GO ORGANIC

Organic dairy products may be good for some people, as well as goat's milk products. In fact, butter in its original form has antimicrobial properties. Coconut oil can have similar antimicrobial effects. When choosing eggs, organic eggs are always a better choice where available. I suspect that exposure to antibiotics in animal foods containing them may play a role in chronic and recurring infections of antibiotic-resistant bacteria.

White flour: The introduction of white flour and sugar caused millions of deaths in isolated primitive races, as discovered by Dr. Weston A. Price in the 1930s. When their previously natural diets were replaced with nutritionally impoverished modern "white" foods, the natural immunity that many races enjoyed suddenly vanished.

Societies that had scarcely seen disease on their native diets were now dying en masse from diseases like tuberculosis and scurvy (vitamin C deficiency). For full coverage of this subject, see the book, *Nutrition and Physical Degeneration* by Weston A. Price, DDS.

In the Australian outback, Dr. Archie Kalokerinos witnessed huge numbers of Australian Aborigine infants dying, and he authored a book on the subject called *Every Second Child*. He eventually discovered that the "white" diet to which they had been recently introduced left them completely malnourished with scurvy (vitamin C deficiency), and hit them especially hard after they were administered vaccines. Aborigine elders lamented to Dr. Kalokerinos, "Before the white man came, we had no disease."[72] (For more on this subject, see the section on vitamin C in the appendix.)

PREVENTING SCURVY

Scurvy is a condition of extreme vitamin C deficiency. Vitamin C is essential for immune function, among other things. Most animals produce vitamin C; humans do not. We must obtain it through our diets. Interestingly, guinea pigs also do not produce vitamin C. This is why these rodents are chosen for laboratory experiments (hence the term "guinea pig" as the quintessential term used to describe an experimental animal).

According to Nobel prize-winning biochemist, Linus Pauling (1901–1994),[73] the recommended daily allowance (RDA) of vitamin C is dangerously low and close to scurvy levels. Most people need between 500–5000 mg of vitamin C every day. While your orange juice container may feature the (bogus) claim that it provides one hundred percent daily value of vitamin C, this is based on the arbitrarily set amount of 60 mg per day. Orange juice is actually *not* a good source vitamin C at all. Vitamin C deteriorates quickly when exposed to air, light, and heat. Orange juice has been subjected to all of these elements by the time it reaches your supermarket refrigerator.

Depending on farming practices, a medium-sized orange may contain anywhere from 0–70 mg of vitamin C. Best-case scenario, you would need to eat about seven *fresh* oranges a day to obtain a minimal 500 mg of vitamin C. Oranges, however, are very mucus producing and are therefore not the best choice for flu season. Other foods that contain lots of vitamin C include bell peppers, kiwis, broccoli, strawberries, cantaloupes, pineapples, cauliflower, and of course, leafy green vegetables.

Our bodies will absorb only as much vitamin C as we need. The rest will be expelled through the bowels. This means that you cannot overdose on vitamin C. Any extra vitamin C will cause harmless and painless diarrhea. During an acute illness, the body can use up its vitamin C

---

72   Archie Kalokerinos, MD, *Every Second Child*, 1974.
73   Linus Pauling, *How to Live Longer and Feel Better*, 1986.

supply rather quickly. Therefore, the best way to take supplemental vitamin C is by splitting it up and taking smaller doses throughout the day, rather than one large dose each day.

VITAMIN D

Another essential immune-building nutrient is vitamin D_3 (chole-calciferol). During the summer, our bodies produce vitamin D when our skin is exposed to sunlight. In the winter, however, it is usually worth supplementing as low sun-exposure levels can lead to vitamin D deficiency, which can result in reduced immune function. During the winter months, it is advisable to supplement with 2000–5000 IU per day of an oil-based vitamin D_3.

EAT RIGHT

In terms of health-promoting foods, fruits and vegetables, nuts and seeds are packed with vitamins and minerals. Dark green leafy vegetables (especially organic) are nutritional superfoods. Also remember to live seasonally. During the winter, drink tea, cook soups, and don't eat cold or iced foods. And, of course, dress appropriately for the weather.

HYGIENE

In terms of hygiene, don't cough or sneeze in other people's faces. I'm sure you knew that already. Of course, it is important to wash your hands, but that probably isn't news to anyone. In fact, I find it remarkable how almost every year we are subjected to news articles reminding us of the importance of hygiene for disease prevention. Perhaps I am mistaken to think that most adults are aware of this bit of common sense. However, be warned that antibacterial soaps have been contributing to antibiotic-resistant super-bacteria, and should be avoided.

I would like to add one more important hygiene caveat. During my clinical internship at a Brooklyn hospital, I worked in a large outpatient center. At the far end of the room was a sink for handwashing. For the convenience of the hospital staff, dispersed throughout the rest of the large area were hand-sanitizer dispensers. Most of the hospital staff availed themselves of the hand sanitizer. I found this practice rather revolting and wondered whether I would want a healthcare provider touching me after touching another patient without washing their hands in between with actual water.

I made my way over to that sink as often as possible, and *always* washed my hands *with water* between patients. With the advent of hand sanitizers, handwashing is becoming a lost art. So I will conclude this section by reminding you that proper hygiene includes washing the dirt *off* of your skin. Many argue that the use of antibacterial hand sanitizers will contribute to the creation and spread of superbugs. Wash your hands with water. And if you observe your healthcare provider using Purell instead of water, you have every right to ask them to wash their hands properly before touching you or your children.

Finally, take two aspirin and call me in the morning. Just kidding.

The following letter was sent to the editor of the magazine when the above article was originally printed.

> *Dear Editor,*
>
> *I feel compelled to offer my opinion. Unfortunately, this past week's article by Yael Tusk, MS, OM, is highly flawed and deserves correction if not retraction. In the article, Yael Tusk makes many assertions about vitamin use, food as medicine, and hand hygiene that are not supported at all by current medical standards and guidelines. Yael Tusk's remarks about hand hygiene are the most potentially dangerous to your readers because they completely contradict federal and international health safety standards.*
>
> *Specifically, she asserts that patients should insist that their healthcare providers wash their hands with soap and water rather than use hand sanitizers, which in her words "contribute to the creation and spread of super-bugs." She ends by cautioning against "Purell" instead of water, and strongly suggests that people insist on having providers wash their hands "properly" before touching the person or her/his children.*

For the record, and the safety of your readers, both the US Centers for Disease Control and Prevention (CDC) and the World Health Organization (WHO) include washing with either an alcohol-based hand sanitizer for twenty to thirty seconds or antimicrobial soap and water for forty to sixty seconds.

Based on meta-analyses of observational studies and randomized controlled trials, one significant problem contributing to nosocomial infections is not the form of hand hygiene the healthcare provider chooses to use, but how long and how thoroughly he or she engages in the hand-hygiene behavior.

In the case of organizations accredited by the Joint Commission, the agency which accredits more than twenty thousand US healthcare organizations, readily accessible alcohol-based products are a requirement for all healthcare workers, not soap and water.

Publishing such a profoundly flawed article runs the risk of harm. The opinion of a single doctor, regardless of how brilliant, doesn't compare to national and international standards that are established after long and rigorous scientific inquiry.

Should you wonder, I am a professional medical publisher who has developed continuing education materials and activities for physicians for the past twenty-five years. I have worked in collaboration with medical school faculty and associations across the country, including Duke, Yale, Harvard, Stanford, Mayo Clinic, Cleveland Clinic, MD Anderson, University of Texas Southwest Health Sciences Center, and many others.

Most sincerely,

D.T.

As D.T. explains, the Centers for Disease Control (CDC) and World Health Organization (WHO) recommend "washing with either an alcohol-based hand sanitizer for 20–30 seconds or antimicrobial soap and water for 40–60 seconds," and asserts that the risk for hospital-acquired infections relates to "not the form of hand hygiene the healthcare provider chooses to use, but how long and how thoroughly he or she engages in the hand-hygiene behavior."

I fully agree with D.T. about the importance of hygiene in a medical setting (or in all settings, for that matter). However, despite its ardent approval by medical authorities, I have serious concerns about the favoring of hand sanitizers over soap and water. While alcohol-based sanitizers are capable of killing many microorganisms, soil can remain on the hands and some microorganisms may survive the process.

Washing with soap and water will remove grime that sanitizers cannot. Even if your healthcare provider has already used a hand sanitizer, washing with running water is definitely in the patient's best interest. What harm could come from washing your hands?

According to D.T., the CDC and WHO are suggesting that real handwashing can be replaced with a thorough rubbing of hand sanitizers on the skin. This protocol is being used in both the medical and food industry.

When it comes to food preparation, hand sanitizers replacing running water is particularly worrisome. Imagine that your friend is hosting you for a meal, and she is preparing a salad for her guests. She notices that her two-year-old needs a diaper change. So your hostess proceeds to change her son's soiled diaper. After disposing of the mess, she pulls a convenient little bottle of hand sanitizer out of her diaper bag, and rubs the liquid on her hands (thoroughly, for a complete thirty seconds)! All the while, there is a sink waiting idle on the other side of the room. She then goes right back to chopping up some tomatoes. How would you feel about eating that salad?

Of course, even when using water, a cursory rinse of the fingertips would be no more beneficial. Obviously, a thorough handwashing is required. Interestingly, according to halachah (Jewish law), one must wash their hands *with water* after using the bathroom or touching any part of the body that is meant to be covered. Where running water is accessible, halachah requires the use of water for handwashing at many times throughout the day.

If hand sanitizers are considered an acceptable alternative to running water, does that mean that hospital and kitchen workers are allowed or encouraged to use hand sanitizers after using the restroom? If yes, then this is truly frightening. If they are not, because this is an obviously unhygienic practice, then why would it be an acceptable way to "wash" between patients?

It is well-known that antibiotic-resistant superbugs are found in every hospital. Even the cleanest looking hospitals can harbor dangerous infectious agents. During my clinical training, I used to rub Purell on my hands, and then follow up with a thorough rinse with running water, when it was available. Could Purell really be adequate to protect the safety of our patients? Today, I would be more hesitant to use a hand sanitizer because of concern about excessive exposure to chemicals. All the more so when these products are used during *food preparation*. These are chemicals that we do not want to eat.

D.T. asserts that my "comments about hand hygiene are the most potentially dangerous to your readers." I cannot fathom what could be dangerous about encouraging washing with soap and running water. If anything, I believe that my suggestion encourages a *higher* level of hygiene than what is required.

So what makes my handwashing suggestions "dangerous"? It would seem that my words, as she puts it, "completely contradict federal and international health safety standards." That by suggesting a different hygiene practice than the currently accepted "standard of care," I am questioning the infallibility of the medical authorities.

Modern medicine is still in its infancy. Despite its technological advancement, medical science still has a long way to go before they have everything figured out. Actually, if they continue with the current reductionist model of the human body (the non-holistic approach; where organs, body parts, and health conditions are diagnosed and treated isolated from the whole, rather than treating the body with an understanding of the interplay between all of all aspects of the human condition), they will *never* figure everything out.

As medical researcher and author Dr. Malcolm Kendrick puts it, *"evidence*-based medicine" has turned into *"eminence*-based medicine". Prestige has turned weak science into hard fact. The credentials of any individual or large medical organization cannot negate common sense. Medical "rules" can and should be subject to individual scrutiny.

I have my reservations about any exciting new medical break-throughs that make the news. Experience has shown that whatever is found safe or true today may be proven dangerous or false tomorrow. With the advent of hand sanitizers, sinks are disappearing from many hospital settings. In their eagerness to embrace the latest innovation, the time-tested method of hygiene is being neglected.

Whenever running water is available, there is good reason to prefer it over chemical or alcohol cleansers. This is true in a medical environment, and even more so when food is involved. There are people who believe that it is dangerous to question the infallibility of the medical authorities. I believe that blind faith in any authority besides our Creator is the real danger.

18

GROUP B
STREP

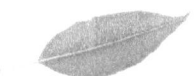

Recently, the GBS (group B strep) test, which is performed on expectant mothers, and the broad use of antibiotics during labor are being questioned by some professionals. When antibiotics are used on millions of asymptomatic (symptom-free) birthing women, we must question whether this is safe, effective, and even necessary.

What is GBS?

Group B strep is a bacterium found in the intestines of many healthy individuals. Infection and illness from GBS does not usually occur, even if it travels to other areas. Having healthy intestinal flora will keep GBS, as well as other disease-causing bacteria, in check.

Since the 1990s, all expectant mothers are tested for GBS between their thirty-fifth to thirty-seventh week. If the test is positive, as it is for 30 percent of women, they will receive IV antibiotics during labor to prevent infection from passing to their newborn. It was once believed that "once GBS, always GBS." In recent years, this has been disproven, as the presence of the bacteria can change in a matter of weeks.

How common is GBS?

Of that 30 percent who test positive for GBS, about one in two hundred mothers who are untreated with antibiotics will deliver a baby who contracts the disease. According to the CDC (Centers for Disease Control), 6 percent of babies infected will die from the illness. This translates to three deaths in ten thousand babies born to GBS positive mothers. This means that ten thousand women have to receive antibiotics to prevent three deadly infections.[74]

A high price to pay — but to save lives, most of us would be willing to do it if antibiotics actually reduced death rates.

According to studies, while antibiotics during labor *may* decrease GBS infection in newborns, there was no decrease in the incidence of death.[75] Why would this be?

Firstly, in the presence of antibiotics, babies are more likely to become infected by drug-resistant bacteria, especially E-coli, which is more deadly than GBS and more difficult to treat, as it is resistant to many antibiotics.[76] [77] Studies have shown that the overall incidence of newborn blood infection and death remained unchanged.[78] One infection may be prevented, while another takes its place.

Why would killing one bacterium cause more harmful bacteria to attack? The answer, I think, is simple: It is not only GBS that is killed by the penicillin, but all the beneficial bacteria that function to keep the E-coli at bay. The antibiotics kill off everything except the resistant strains, which are then able to flourish and cause harm.

---

74   "Treating Group B Strep: Are Antibiotics Necessary?" Mothering Editorial, last updated 09/30/10.

75   Ibid.

76   C.V. Towers, M.H. Carr, G. Padilla, T. Asrat. J. Am, Obstet Gynecol, "Potential consequences of widespread antepartal use of ampicillin," University of California, Irvine, USA. 1998 Oct;179(4):879–83, http://www.ncbi.nlm.nih.gov/pubmed/9790363.

77   E. M. Levine, V. Ghai, J. J. Barton, and C. M. Strom, "Intrapartum Antibiotic Prophylaxis Increases the Incidence of Gram-Negative Neonatal Sepsis," *Infectious Diseases in Obstetrics and Gynecology*, Volume 7 (1999), Issue 4, Pages 210–213.

78   "Treating Group B Strep: Are Antibiotics Necessary?" Mothering Editorial.

Premature infants are at greater risk of contracting GBS. However, they are also much more susceptible to infection from super-bacteria triggered by antibiotics. Severe complications, even deaths, have occurred in premature infants when women whose waters broke before thirty-seven weeks were given antibiotics to prevent GBS.[79]

Since the initiation of administering antibiotics to millions of women during labor, studies have shown that some strains of GBS are becoming resistant to all forms of antibiotics as well.[80] The CDC openly states in its literature that antibiotics are only a temporary solution because of drug resistance.[81]

In addition, an NIH study of newborns who tested positive for GBS, whose mothers received penicillin during labor, had three times more respiratory distress within two days of birth when compared with GBS-positive newborns of untreated mothers. Studies have also shown that antibiotics given during pregnancy are associated with greater incidence of allergies and asthma in children.[82]

Is there anything else that can be done to prevent GBS before going into labor?

- As mentioned above, healthy bacterial flora can keep harmful bacteria in check. Consider taking probiotics, or use a fermented food like sauerkraut.
- A diet high in complex carbohydrates (whole grains) and lots of vegetables and fruit have been shown to help maintain healthy bacteria.
- Garlic has been proven to have strong antibacterial qualities.[83]

---

79   Ibid.
80   Ibid.
81   Cohain, J.S.; "Newborn Group B Strep Infection: Top 10 Reasons to Not Culture at 36 Weeks," *Midwifery Today*, 2010.
82   Ibid.
83   Cohain, J.S., CNM, "How to Treat a Vaginal Infection with a Clove of Garlic," *Midwifery Today*, 2007, http://www.midwiferytoday.com/articles/garlic.asp See article for instructions.

In the hospital:

- Receiving many internal examinations (over six) is a known risk factor for transmitting GBS.
- Avoid artificial rupture of membranes, as this may also increase the chance of infection.[84]
- Keep hands really clean, and keep your newborn from being exposed to too many hands. GBS and other infections can be transmitted outside the womb, and hospitals are notorious sources of many resistant bacteria.

My advice to mothers is to labor at home for as long as possible to reduce the dangers to both mother and baby.

According to the CDC, antibiotics should only be used when strictly necessary. The current prophylactic use of antibiotics on 10–30 percent of birthing women worldwide is hard to justify in light of the CDC's grave concerns about antibiotic resistance.

---

84   Cohain, J.S., "Newborn Group B Strep Infection: Top 10 Reasons to Not Culture at 36 Weeks," *Midwifery Today*, 2010.

19

CHILDBIRTH

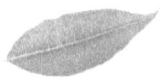

Women are in labor longer today than in previous generations. Women used to be told that a first birth takes an average of twelve hours, and subsequent labors are averaged at six hours. Strangely, in recent years, these numbers have doubled! Today, women are laboring for time periods that are longer than ever before. It is now the norm for a woman to labor for longer than twenty-four hours!

Some creative medical thinkers have opined that prolonged labor can be a good thing, as it gives doctors more time to intervene. This is preposterous, since if these women's labors would have progressed more quickly, they would never have needed intervention in the first place. Most women are aware that they are infinitely better off in terms of their own health and the safety of their baby if their labor and birth occur naturally.

Woman was created to give birth naturally, without the assistance of modern-day interventions. Why are so many women in labor today experiencing a shutdown? "Failure to progress" is the vague term used to describe any labor that is taking longer than the established norms. Sometimes contractions become ineffective, or stop altogether.

Ideally, if the labor stops, the woman should be left alone and allowed to rest. *Labor will start on its own when the body is ready.* In today's hospital settings, women are rarely allowed this luxury. In response to a slowed labor, often even in the absence of fetal distress, medical intervention is commonly used. This can lead to a cascade: from anesthesia to induction, to vacuum, forceps, and surgery.

Although anesthesia is not risk free, it is always used in surgery since it would be impossible to tolerate surgical pain. The same line of reasoning has been transferred to using anesthesia in childbirth. The commonly held belief is that labor pain is unbearable, making anesthesia seemingly indispensable.

Why is it that women are experiencing increasingly traumatic labors today? And what causes labor to shut down, resulting in the high level of medical intervention?

In Western society, childbirth has become a dramatic affair. It seems that the advent of epidurals has created an extreme fear of labor. Once the pain of labor can be turned off, experiencing the sensation seems much more unbearable. Additionally, because many labor and delivery wards have an air of an emergency room in which childbirth is treated like a life-threatening illness, the situation is made much more frightening than it needs to be.

Women from primitive villages with little or no exposure to the media give birth without assistance calmly and easily. No drama, no complications; it's all they know. When women go into labor without fear, the birth process will usually run a lot more smoothly. The notion that labor has to be excruciating is a modern invention. It is tension and fear of childbirth that actually *cause* mothers to experience unbearable labors.

HOW FEAR AFFECTS LABOR

During labor, a woman may naturally become fearful. This fear causes the body to react with the stress/fight-or-flight response, where the body is readied for an emergency. In an unconscious defensive effort, the body will try to prevent the birth from progressing until the emergency state has passed. So stress and fear can invariably lead to failure to progress. Natural, unconscious instincts will not allow the body to give birth until it feels safe once again.

While childbirth may naturally cause discomfort, what we are experiencing today is a *malfunction in the birth process, as is evident in the increasing lengths of labors today*. When there is fear, the muscles that are meant to relax and open remain tense and tightly closed. This causes contractions to be very painful and ineffective. This kind of pain is anything but a natural part of childbirth.

THE POWER OF RELAXATION

If an expectant mother goes into labor relaxed and calm, without fear, the birthing muscles will work in harmony and with ease. It is no wonder that labor often starts in the middle of the night, when the mother is sleeping. The body is in an ultra-relaxed state, when it can do its job naturally and easily without any interference from our active, nervous minds.

Having the right tools can make childbirth a wonderful experience.

When trying to relax, especially during a challenging situation like childbirth, many discover that they are incapable of doing so. This problem can be resolved when expectant mothers learn how to use effective relaxation methods. These techniques allow us to regain control of our minds, and stop letting tension negatively affect the labor process. With proper training, *anyone* can learn to relax and allow labor to progress naturally.

Women who learn to use these tools for childbirth often have significantly shorter and less painful births. Many women who have given birth previously with some difficulty have reported that after taking a course in deep relaxation or hypnosis for childbirth, their birth experience was transformed into a serene and wonderful one.

BETTER BIRTH OUTCOMES

Mothers who are trained in relaxation are much less likely to need medical intervention. While some women would prefer an epidural, things don't always work out as planned. Often, a woman (usually not a first-time mother) will enter the hospital intent on getting her epidural, only to discover that she has progressed too far to receive one; i.e., birth is imminent.

Some may call this a blessing, and others a curse. Regardless of how you feel about a quick labor, having something up your sleeve that is not dependent on outside circumstances is undeniably helpful. It is also noteworthy that babies born to mothers who used relaxation or hypnosis during labor tend to be calmer, and adjust more easily to life outside the womb. Women who have a great birth experience also experience easier recovery after birth and less postpartum depression.

OVERDUE?

Shoshana scheduled an appointment at my clinic for an acupuncture induction. In my office, she explained that she was thirty-seven weeks, and expecting twins. A recent ultrasound indicated that one of the babies was smaller than the other, as compared to a previous ultrasound, so the doctor told her to go for an immediate induction. He explained that the smaller baby was receiving less nutrition and was therefore in danger.

Becky came to my office for an appointment for an induction. She was only thirty-eight weeks, but the ultrasound showed that amniotic fluid was low and the placenta was old. She told me that according to her friends, the doctor who performed her ultrasound was the best in the city.

Shaina came in reporting that the ultrasound showed that her baby was 4.1 kg at thirty-eight weeks. The doctor warned her that it would be dangerous to wait for labor to commence naturally, because who knew how big the baby would be by then?

After consulting with me and other childbirth experts, doulas, etc., all three of the above women decided to wait on the recommended induction. All of their babies were born naturally without any evidence of the problems reported via ultrasound. This is because ultrasounds are notoriously unreliable. Going for an induction based on ultrasound alone will usually lead to unnecessary intervention.

Medical inductions can endanger the mother and baby, and I advise women to evaluate whether it is the right decision to attempt to bring the baby into this world before it's ready. In most cases, labor will start when the baby is ready to be born, and not a moment sooner.

Ultrasounds have led to a lot more intervention, yet they have not improved health outcome when compared to babies who were not constantly monitored.

If induction *is* indicated, try any and every natural method first. Unlike Pitocin or prostaglandins, which can make labor more painful and unregulated and often lead to further invasive interventions, acupuncture is a risk-free method of induction. Rather than aggressively overriding the body's natural responses, it gently strengthens and stimulates them. Women who receive acupuncture before labor usually have easier and quicker labors, and rarely end up in surgery.

I perform acupuncture inductions all the time, and the success rate is quite high. But unless there is an urgent medical reason, I rarely perform them before thirty-nine weeks (thirty-eight weeks for twins). Once a woman has reached forty weeks, I will use acupuncture to induce with no questions asked.

NATURAL METHODS FOR INDUCTION

It is not necessary to automatically go for an induction just because you are post-date. As I mentioned above, barring unique circumstances, induction, even via natural means, should be reserved for full-term babies (i.e., forty weeks). The following are some of the safer techniques to bring on labor.

- **Walking** — Anyone who's taken my childbirth class knows that I discourage excessive exercise during labor and favor rest and relaxation. To bring on labor, however, walking or exercise may help. Don't exhaust yourself, and make sure to rest as well. You'll need your strength later.
- **Rest and Relaxation** — For some women, the only reason they go post-date is because of tension. They may actually be fighting labor. Don't wait until you are post-date to deal with fear and tension. Relaxation can be accomplished with the help of hypnosis, guided imagery, acupuncture, or with a trip to a spa.
- **Evening Primrose Oil** — A popular remedy among doulas, known to soften the cervix. It may be taken orally (I can't vouch for kashrus) or locally. It should not be used for VBACs.

- **Red Raspberry Leaf Tea** — Strengthening and full of essential nutrients. Can be taken the entire third trimester, and even postpartum. As you approach your due date, you can increase the dose from one cup to three cups per day.
- **Castor Oil** — I've never personally recommended this one, since I've heard too many reports of it instigating painful diarrhea. However, some women swear by it. It doesn't cause pain for everyone. Use under the guidance of a doula.
- **High Dose Vitamin C** — Peristalsis seems to induce contractions for many women. High doses of ascorbic acid can loosen the bowels and therefore may bring on labor. But unlike castor oil, it should be painless.
- **Homeopathy** — Remedies vary according to the individual's constitution. Must be matched for each person with the help of a natural-health practitioner or homeopath.
- **Black and Blue Cohosh** — Use only when you're full term! These can cause miscarriage if taken in the first or second trimester. Use under the supervision of an experienced herbalist.
- **Acupuncture** — Very safe, though you can't do it yourself. Can induce labor, shorten the length of labor, and reduce the chance of needing other interventions. Sometimes, more than one visit is necessary, though for many women, one treatment is all it takes to get labor going.
- **Reflexology** — Also very safe. Many women see good results from a treatment or two.

None of these methods will work for everyone, and there is good reason to try as many of them as possible (except castor oil, which I'd save for last).

See appendix B for solutions for breech babies.

20

NEWBORN
HEALTHCARE

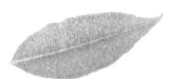

A couple of years ago, I overheard a conversation between two women sitting next to me at a social gathering. One of the women mentioned that she left the hospital right after her baby was born. When she told the hospital staff that she wanted to leave, they put up quite a fight. After she received her release papers, a pediatric nurse, who was among those pushing her to stay, approached her and quietly said, "Between you and me, the hospital is the worst place for a newborn. I also leave as soon as I can!" She worked in the nursery, so she knew firsthand.

Aside from understaffed and overcrowded nurseries, babies are administered a lot of medication during their first few days of life. I always had my reservations about these preventative interventions. Not knowing the true benefits or risks of these procedures prompted me to do a lot of research so that I could make more educated decisions.

Many people believe that whatever intervention modern medicine has to offer can be only beneficial. This is simply not true. In fact, a huge number of interventions performed today are not based on sound scientific evidence; findings often contradict the procedures.

In the childbirth classes I give, I have observed that many mothers share my concern about the risks they are exposing their newborns to. So for the sake of all future infants (whose parents read this book), I am sharing here the fruits of my research so that you can make informed decisions, should you desire to do so.

Here is a list of some commonly performed hospital procedures that your newborn will invariably be exposed to, including their purpose, as well as the risks involved.

Antibiotic Eye Ointment

This procedure is used to prevent chlamydia and gonorrhea infection from passing to the baby's eyes. Gonorrhea is a bacterial infection that is sexually transmitted. If there is any reason to suspect that the mother is infected, she can be tested. In other words, your baby is unnecessarily given a preventative treatment for an infection that mother can easily be screened for.

The risks of this treatment appear to be low, and include eye irritation and blurred vision. Excessive use of antibiotics may also contribute to the development of antibiotic-resistant bacteria. Balance this against the fact that the benefits, for most babies, amount to zero if the mother is not infected.[85]

Hepatitis B Vaccine

Hepatitis B is a rare viral infection. It is spread through blood and body fluids (not sneezes), and primarily affects IV drug users and promiscuous individuals. It is rarely found in children. The only babies who are at risk of contracting hepatitis B are those whose mothers carry the disease, or in the unlikely event that they receive a blood transfusion from an infected donor. The vaccine has been administered to infants less than a day old since 1991.

---

85   Rebecca Dekker, PhD, RN, APRN. "Is Erythromycin Eye Ointment Always Necessary for Newborns?" 2012.

Why are babies given this vaccine?

The vaccine manufacturers admit that they give the shot to babies because they were unsuccessful in accessing the population actually at risk of contracting the disease! In the words of GlaxoSmithKline, infants are vaccinated for hepatitis B "because a vaccination strategy limited to high-risk individuals has failed,"[86] and children are "accessible."[87] So, in essence, most infants are exposed to the risks of a vaccine for a disease irrelevant to them, ostensibly to protect IV drug users, etc.

Hepatitis B is another disease where the mother can easily be screened during pregnancy for the presence of infection. It is less invasive to screen mothers for the disease than to inject billions of babies without regard to the mother's infection status.

"I'd rather not put up a fight — can't I just let them do it anyway?"

I mentioned the above information during a childbirth class that I was teaching. One mother called me after the birth of her baby to tell me the great news. She mentioned that her husband did not want to fight the medical staff, and preferred to take the vaccine.

Not every hospital will give you a hard time if you choose to reject this injection. However, even if they do give you trouble, you might decide that it is still worth it. Consider the following: The National Vaccine Information Center has received reports of many adverse reactions to this vaccine, including severe dermatological disease, seizures, arthritis, autoimmune disorders, diabetes, and infant death. According to researcher J. Barthelow Classen, MD, the vaccine causes approximately ten thousand cases of diabetes in the US each year.

When information from the US government's Vaccine Adverse Event Reporting System was analyzed, the number of serious adverse reactions to the vaccine in children, *by far* outnumbered cases of the disease.[88] In 1993, *Pediatrics* magazine reported that according to surveys,

---

86   GlaxoSmithKline Biologicals. Engerix-B [Hepatitis B vaccine (recombinant)]. Product insert (December 2006).

87   Schaffner W, Gardner P, Gross PA. "Hepatitis B immunization strategies: expanding the target," *Annals of Internal Medicine* (Feb 15, 1993); 118(4): 308–309.

88   Miller, Neil Z. *Vaccine Safety Manual for Concerned Families and Health Practitioners*, 2010, p. 91.

up to eighty-seven percent of pediatricians did not believe that the vaccine was appropriate for their newborn patients. (The results would likely be different today, as the vaccine's administration has become so widespread that doctors have probably forgotten who is truly at risk of contracting this disease.)

Immune Suppression

Despite what is commonly believed, vaccines act as immunosuppressants. An infant's immune system takes about three years to develop fully. The changes made during these early developmental stages can have lifelong ramifications. In the short run, this injection, among others, can threaten the immune system's ability to deal with other foreign invasions, possibly rendering innocuous microorganisms deadly. Depressing an infant's immature immune system is a dangerous game. In the long run, the possible harm is unknown, because long-term studies on this vaccine have never been done!

Vitamin K Injection

It is believed that one in ten thousand babies have some form of bleeding during the first few weeks of life due to vitamin K deficiency. In just over five out of one hundred thousand infants, bleeding in the brain occurs, usually three to seven weeks after birth. Forty percent of these infants suffer permanent brain damage or death. Bleeding in the brain is usually a result of undetected liver disease, where the liver is unable to manufacture blood-clotting factors out of vitamin K. Infants exposed to drugs or alcohol are at the greatest risk of liver disease. Babies have a higher risk of bleeding if their mothers took medications, including antibiotics and epileptic drugs, while expecting.

Additional vitamin K will help these five children. That is why hospitals routinely give this injection. However, some studies show that injecting a dose of vitamin K that is twenty thousand times the newborn level may cause an 80 percent increased risk of developing childhood leukemia. "Extracting data from available literature reveals that there are 1.5 extra cases of leukemia per one hundred thousand children due to vitamin K injections, and 1.8 more permanent injuries or deaths per one hundred thousand, due to brain bleeding without injections."[89]

Further research uncovered that the injection given in the hospital contains other ingredients aside from a megadose of vitamin K. Depending on the manufacturer, it may contain hydrochloric acid, aluminum, or benzyl alcohol, which have been associated with toxicity in newborns. According to package inserts, "Hyperbilirubinemia [jaundice] has occurred in newborns following the administration of vitamin K injection." The vitamin K shot, which contains legume oil, may be one of the causes of the modern-day peanut-allergy epidemic. More on this later.

Since vitamin K is fat soluble, overdose may be more easily achieved. Though the risk may not be high, there is reason to be concerned, since vitamin K overdose can cause anaphylaxis, liver damage, and brain damage — which is of particular concern for the developing infant brain.[90]

Despite all these risks, the numbers seem to favor vitamin K supplementation. However, there are other options aside from a huge overdose through a (possibly dangerous) injection at birth:

- **Formula** is supplemented with large doses of vitamin K, making supplementation by injection unnecessary for formula-fed infants. (For the record, I do not advocate formula, unless unusual circumstances necessitate it.)
- Interestingly, **colostrum** (first milk) contains larger amounts of vitamin K than the milk that follows. One study found that infants who were allowed unrestricted nursing during their first twenty-four hours of life did not suffer from bleeding.[91] Other researchers found that mother's milk has the highest levels of vitamin K on days seven and eight after birth, right around the time of circumcision!

89   Linda Folden Palmer, DC, International Chiropractic Pediatric Association Newsletter, September/October 2002 Issue, updated May 19, 2004.

90   Reed Group, Medical Disability Advisor, "Poisoning, Vitamin K," 2012. http://www.md-guidelines.com/poisoning-vitamin-k.

91   Joanna Karpasea-Jones, "Vitamin K: Does Your Baby Really Need It? Vitamin K Injection: Is it really just a vitamin?" *The Mother Magazine*.

- For babies who nurse and did not receive the shot at birth, if the mother is concerned, she can take a one-milligram vitamin K supplement daily for ten weeks. This will provide a cumulative extra one milligram to her infant over that crucial period. Or the infant can be given a low oral dose of two hundred micrograms of liquid vitamin K_9, once a week for five weeks, totaling one milligram.[92]

TAKE CARE OF YOUR HEALTH

It is rare for health to spontaneously malfunction (to an extreme degree) in infants in the absence of some sort of provocation. In reality, when illness occurs, causative factors are often present. In Chinese medicine, there is an understanding that disease is the result of some sort of deficiency or excess, which can be understood here as nutritional deficiencies or excess toxins.

The best way to ensure a healthy baby is for the mother to eat well and avoid unnecessary pharmaceutical drugs and other toxins during pregnancy. While problems may arise despite our best efforts, they do not usually occur unprovoked. Therefore, there is reason to believe that babies are born whole and healthy. The current focus on obscure health defects and the prophylactic treatment of all infants for potential disease undermines a mother's belief in her ability to naturally care for and provide nutrition for her infant both before and after birth.

The best way to ensure a healthy baby is through good nutrition. Note that nursing mothers will have more vitamin K if they consume leafy green vegetables. Other sources of vitamin K include scallions, prunes (watch out for preservatives), cucumbers, dried basil, and broccoli.[93] True preventative medicine means taking care of your health to prevent illness from occurring in the first place.

There is a widespread yet mistaken notion that only professionals are capable of understanding health issues and treatments. The truth

---

92   Linda Folden Palmer, DC, "Vitamin K at Birth: To Inject or Not?" International Chiropractic Pediatric Association Newsletter, September/October 2002 Issue, updated May 19, 2004.

93   Dr. Josh Axe, "Top 10 Vitamin K Rich Foods," https://draxe.com/top-10-vitamin-k-rich-foods/.

is that every medical consumer will be better off if they understand what they are being offered and why, and only then make an educated decision. Before taking any medication, read the package insert. If you see side effects that disturb you, don't brush them aside as rare complications. Ask yourself: Do the benefits truly outweigh the risks? Is this drug potentially more harmful than the ailment it is treating?

When it comes to your own health, and even more so when it comes to your children's health, a bit of educated skepticism is in order. Those who are well-informed are able to differentiate between harmful and beneficial treatments, and will have a basis upon which to choose to either accept or reject offered treatments.

21

LACTATION

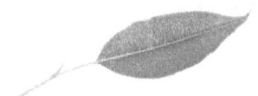

Half a century ago, in a (highly successful) effort to market their products, formula manufacturers claimed that their milk substitutes were better than mother's milk. Society took the bait, and nursing fell out of favor. The tantalizing freedom that mothers gained, since bottle-feeding could be accomplished by just about anyone, has left its mark. Mothers the world over were suddenly able to leave even the tiniest infants in the care of others, in order to return to work.

Thankfully, the situation has recently reversed, and nursing is once again recognized as the ideal choice for infants. In many communities, nursing is once again "in vogue." Today, many working mothers try to supply their own milk, but often the long separation causes milk supply to dwindle rapidly.

Society is in a sorry state today, where in many circles a "stay-at-home mom" has become an object of ridicule. The truth is that being a full-time mother is a very noble job, and mothers who choose this path deserve great respect. They are working harder than anyone.

On the other hand, there are many women who want to nurse, but for various reasons end up giving up. For the most part, lactation failure can be ascribed to seemingly (and sometimes genuinely) insurmountable nursing challenges or insufficient milk supply.

TIPS TO INCREASE MILK SUPPLY

- Nurse on demand. Babies will not keep to a one-size-fits-all nursing schedule. When your baby seems hungry, feed him. Do not push him off, even if the clock says it's too soon to nurse again. This is especially true in the first few weeks of life. (On the other hand, if the baby is crying after having just nursed, it is unlikely that he needs to be fed again — look for other possible causes of crying, such as tiredness, constipation, or indigestion.)
- Do not try to train your infant to sleep through the night, especially if milk supply is an issue.
- Since you should not expect your baby to follow a rigid schedule, do not wake him up to nurse. If he is sleeping, that's what he needs to do. He will wake up on his own when he is hungry. No baby ever died of starvation in their sleep. Babies are at their most instinctual phase of their lives. You can rest assured: his body knows what it needs, and you can follow those cues.
- Don't give your baby a pacifier when he's hungry! This is a surefire way to interfere with the message to produce more milk.
- Give your baby as much time as he needs to nurse. As long as baby is actively sucking, do not try to minimize feeding time, relying on arbitrary numbers.
- Eat, eat, and eat. Lactating mothers should never limit calorie consumption. This can starve your baby. Do not prioritize your own weight loss over your infant's weight gain.
- Certain foods can improve milk supply, including carrots, carp, red meat, and fatty foods. If you eat dairy, choose full-fat first.
- Take herbal remedies that boost milk production, such as fennel and fenugreek.
- If insufficient milk is an issue for you, avoid being separated from your baby. Do not leave the baby with a sitter with a bottle of formula; this will only decrease your milk supply.

- Do not supplement with formula unless you have exhausted all other resources for producing adequate milk.
- Pump for at least ten minutes after nursing to give your body the message to produce more milk.
- If the baby's suck is not good, consider trying craniosacral therapy treatment.

To be certain that your baby is receiving enough milk, check for frequent wet diapers. Also look at overall weight gain, energy level, mood, and satiety after nursing. If you have the occasion to pump when the baby has not recently eaten, you should be able to produce at least three to four ounces of milk.

NO MILK?

In more than one book on nursing, I have seen authors describe low or no milk supply as a total impossibility, and a challenge that can always be overcome. They advise to keep working on methods to stimulate lactation with the belief that all women can nurse, and that failure to produce adequate milk can only be due to a lack of effort on the mother's part.

This is dangerous advice, and, in my experience, is not based on reality. In cases where things are just not working no matter what is attempted, this advice can lead to a starving infant and a guilt-ridden mother who believes that despite giving it her all, she must be doing something wrong since the milk is not coming.

While it is unusual to be totally unable to lactate, there are cases where women cannot produce milk, no matter how hard they try. I have seen this happen particularly in women with health conditions like hypothyroidism and polycystic ovary syndrome. This is by no means an across-the-board phenomenon. Plenty of women with these diagnoses can nurse successfully. However, some cannot no matter how hard they try, or they may produce some milk, but not enough to completely satisfy their infant's needs.

If despite your best efforts the milk does not arrive, it may be through no fault of your own, but may be the result of a systemic imbalance that makes supplementation necessary. On too many occasions, I have seen lactation advocates write that all women can nurse successfully if they make a concerted effort, and this is simply not the case! While it always good to try, if you've given it your best effort and no milk is forthcoming, don't blame yourself. Sometimes a health problem simply prevents adequate — or any — lactation. Just because lactation works for most people, that does not mean it will work for everyone.

For most women, lactation becomes the most special time to bond with their infant and relax (and sit!). Even if one has no choice but to bottle-feed, mothers can still treat feedings as sacred — take the baby to a quiet room and sit in a comfortable chair, cuddle the baby close, and the baby may get nearly as much out of the bottle as he would if he nursed.

INTRODUCING SOLIDS

During the past few years, parents have been introducing solid foods to their infants at increasingly younger ages. Traditionally, babies nursed exclusively for *at least* the first six months of life. Yet some mothers have begun giving solid foods to infants under four months of age. This is a problem; there is agreement across the board in all medical traditions that a newborn's digestive system is extremely underdeveloped and cannot handle anything besides mother's milk during the first half a year after birth.

A recent CDC study found that babies who were fed formula exclusively were most likely to be introduced to solids prematurely, whereas infants who were exclusively nursed were least likely. Surveys indicated that the reason formula-fed babies tend to receive food earlier is the prohibitive cost of formula versus the cheapness and convenience of readily available food.

While six months is the earliest safe age to begin solid foods, this may be too young for some children. As long as the child is satisfied with nursing and developing well, there is no reason to rush to introduce food. In my experience, babies often begin to suffer from digestive problems after solid foods have been introduced. Common reactions to solids include allergies, constipation, diarrhea, digestive discomfort, gassiness, and pain. These are signs that the baby's digestive tract is not yet ready for what you are giving him. If this happens to your child, revert to the previous feeding pattern, and wait for his digestion to return to normal before trying new foods again.[94]

Before rushing to introduce food to your infant, remember — mother's milk contains everything your baby needs.

If insufficient milk supply is the motivation to introduce solids, first consider taking supplements that boost lactation. These include herbs, such as fennel, fenugreek, or an herbal formula prescribed by a professional herbalist, as well as a variety of foods. Barley malt is a particularly effective milk booster found in beer and black beer, which is alcohol free. Other foods include carrot, sweet potato, carp, chicken, black sesame seeds, and roasted peanuts.

When introducing solid foods to a nursing infant, consider the first few weeks to be purely practice for your baby. It really doesn't matter if nothing is swallowed if the child is receiving nourishment from nursing.

In addition to waiting until there is a genuine need to start solids, be careful to start with foods that are relatively bland and easily digested, such as single grains, well-cooked vegetables, and chicken soup. I heard of one young couple who decided that avocado would be a good first food for their child. Initially, they considered the endeavor a huge success, since the infant ate half an avocado his first time around. The child proceeded to vomit the entire thing. While avocado is a popular and highly nutritious baby food, it is extremely heavy and rich, and should only be given to a seasoned eater.

Teething trouble is caused primarily by digestive disturbance, so the richer a baby's diet, and the more digestive difficulty there is, the more likely they are to suffer from teething pain. By giving your child a bland, easily digestible diet, you may avoid many sleepless nights.

Not to worry; it will not be long before your child is eating adult foods along with everyone else. Just wait until his digestive system has had sufficient time to practice with foods that are easier to process. There is no limit to the number of ailments that can be avoided by careful weaning.

---

94   If the situation does not improve even after simplifying the diet, acupuncture treatment may be helpful to "reset" the system.

Remember:

- Do not begin solids before six months.
- Boost lactation before giving up on nursing in favor of solids.
- To keep up milk supply, nurse regularly while introducing solids.
- Don't rush to wean. Continue to nurse throughout this process to avoid being excessively dependent on the foods introduced, since babies may spit out all solid foods for a while before getting the hang of it.
- The later you introduce solids, the less likely your infant will suffer from digestive disturbance or teething trouble.
- For the same reason, introduce bland foods first.
- Don't sweeten unnecessarily to entice your baby. As long as you're nursing, the baby is getting nourishment. Persist with unsweetened choices as long as possible since it is preferable that the child does not develop a sweet tooth too young.

22

COLIC

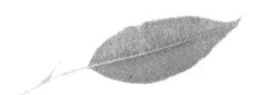

Why do infants have such sensitive stomachs? Even if they are not suffering from constant colic, as so many babies do, most babies still seem to have a tendency toward digestive disturbances, such as abdominal pain (and the constant crying that tends to go with it), constipation, diarrhea, and excessive regurgitating.

Even if the nursing mother tries to eat very carefully, it still seems that the slightest provocation can cause an infant's digestion to go haywire. Why are their stomachs so much more sensitive than their adult counterparts?

A newborn's digestive tract is very immature, and still must undergo much development. Despite the inexperience, this immature system is immediately demanded to digest enough food to double the infant's body weight in a mere few months' time. An infant's digestive system is comparable to a major city highway at rush hour, where the slightest incident can cause miles of bumper-to-bumper traffic in all directions.

The amount of food a tiny infant's GI tract must process and integrate is enormous in proportion to its minute size. If a ten-pound baby consumes four ounces of milk, imagine the equivalent in an adult weighing 120 pounds. It would mean consuming forty-eight ounces (six cups) in one sitting! It's no wonder that an infant's immature digestive system can become so quickly overloaded. So it becomes more apparent how the slightest provocation can then lead to the entire digestive system shutting down and creating the immense discomfort that ensues.

There are those who argue that digestive health depends on the infant's inheritance of gut flora at birth.[95] Some postulate that cesarean section causes infants to bypass the natural pathway toward "microbiome" inheritance. (The microbiome is made up of trillions of microbes — bacteria, fungi, and more — living within the human body, especially the gut, that play an important role in both health and sickness.) Although I am convinced that C-sections are not beneficial to infant health, I am somewhat skeptical that birth is the only opportunity to absorb gut bacteria, and suspect that it is a much longer and more complex process with lots of ups and downs along the way. Nevertheless, I suspect that infants whose mothers received antibiotics during pregnancy or who received antibiotics after birth are at greater risk of suffering from digestive disturbance, which may very well be due to chronic gut-flora imbalance.

Usually, in cases of genuine colic, there will be symptoms of irregular digestion, which may include one or more of the following:

- Less frequent bowel movements or skipped days (see chapter on constipation for more on this — once a week is *not* enough)
- Signs of straining or discomfort before bowel movements
- Mucus in the stool
- Strangely colored stools, such as orange, green, or brown (nursing infants' stools should be yellow)
- Consistent screaming after meals
- Excessive spit-up, especially when accompanied by mucus
- Spit-up that smells foul

What can be done to make our infant's digestion run as smoothly as possible? It is now well-known and widely accepted that mother's

---

95   Natasha Campbell McBride, MD, *Gut and Psychology Syndrome: Natural Treatment for Autism, ADD/ADHD, Dyslexia, Dyspraxia*, 2004.

milk is the ideal choice for infants. We are also aware of the importance of the mother maintaining an optimal diet and testing and avoiding trigger foods (such as dairy, coffee, chocolate, cabbage, beans, spicy foods, and possibly wheat). Eliminating potential trigger foods can be attempted one at a time and kept up for at least two weeks, while observing changes. As the baby grows and gets happier, trigger foods may be cautiously reintroduced.

What can be done if, despite our best efforts, an infant is still not tolerating mother's milk?

There are a few natural home remedies for colic, some of which originate in Chinese medicine:

- Roasted rice tea — when mother's milk is not tolerated, roast one part rice in a skillet until it is dark brown. Then add three parts water and simmer for twenty minutes, and then pour off the tea. Give your infant a few ounces once or twice daily.
- Chew a bag of green tea and then place it in your infant's belly button and cover it with a Band-Aid. Let it remain in place for a few hours.
- One remedy that a colleague of mine swears by is to rub warm olive oil on the infant's abdomen and then wrap the abdomen in a cloth diaper.
- I have personally found acupuncture to be extremely helpful in relieving many cases of colic; sometimes, just a few treatments are enough to bring about long-term relief, making other actions unnecessary.

Mother's milk is in a class of its own and cannot be replaced with any formula. If the baby still cannot tolerate mother's milk, or if it is not available, the following are the next-best options:

- Goat's milk (preferably organic) works well, though it should not be used alone. Goats are very clean animals and they graze on a much wider variety of plants than do their bovine counterparts, which makes their milk much higher in nutritional content. In addition, the fat structure in goat's milk is far more digestible than cow's milk. Also, because of this fat structure, goat's milk is homogeneous in its natural state, which means that it is not necessary to subject it to the harmful[96] homogenization process. Most infants tolerate goat's milk well, even those who cannot tolerate mother's milk and cow's milk.

- The next choice is a high-quality infant formula.
- The *last* choice is unhomogenized organic cow's milk.

Some pediatricians have argued that animal milk is unsafe for infants under a year old. I find this rather mysterious since it is an ingredient in any dairy infant formula. The main issue with cow's milk is that it may be allergenic or difficult to digest. This problem is not always solved when it is put in formula. In my years treating children with colic, I've come across children who are allergic to mother's milk and even hypoallergenic formulas. If these children are able to digest goat's milk, then this option should be considered, because it's certainly preferred to starvation. Only a baby who is allergic to goat's milk needs to avoid it.

Synthetic infant formulas have a track record for occasionally lacking certain essential nutrients. A look at international history reveals that in many instances, formulas produced that inadvertently lacked nutrients subsequently led to malnutrition with deadly ramifications. As recently as February 2016, there was a recall of Nestle brand infant formula in Canada because it lacked certain essential minerals. Formulas also carry a risk of being contaminated with heavy metals and microorganisms.

Since there is no perfect replacement to mother's milk, when mother's milk is not available, it is safest to combine substitutes to prevent malnutrition. Goat's milk alone may not adequately replace mother's milk, and is best when combined with other options, as in goat's milk plus a quality infant formula, or expressed donor's milk. Nutritional supplements may also be necessary.

---

96   It is best to avoid homogenized milk because the process breaks down certain enzymes (which are normally excreted during digestion) into tiny shards, which then readily pass into the bloodstream unhindered and accumulate in the blood vessels, possibly even causing vascular degeneration. (P. Pitchford, *Healing with Whole Foods*).

When a substitute is given, it is important that the milk be warmed. One should not give a baby food or milk directly from the refrigerator. Not only can cold food dramatically weaken an infant's already tender digestive system, but it may even trigger colic. In order for digestion to work efficiently, the food must be at body temperature. Cold foods will force your baby to unnecessarily expend a tremendous amount of digestive energy in order to bring the food to an ideal temperature.

WHEN IT'S NOT REALLY COLIC

Keep in mind that one of the most common causes of inconsolable screaming in infants may not be colic at all, but may really be the result of vaccination, which can cause pain and inflammation in the gut, brain, and many other organ systems. I used to believe that colic was almost always really a mislabeled vaccine reaction, but I have come to discover that colic exists even among my unvaccinated infant patients. It is easier to differentiate between genuine colic and an inflammatory vaccine reaction when vaccines are delayed or in babies that are unvaccinated.

I am particularly concerned that since the hepatitis B vaccine is given only a few hours after birth, mothers may never really see what their infant's health would have looked like unmedicated. From day one, as soon as the process of pharmaceutical disease prevention begins, it becomes difficult to differentiate between a genuine intrinsic health problem and one that was instigated by an outside force.

Colic is a very common condition, but I hope parents can find solace in the fact that one day soon, the infant will grow out of it (unless, of course, it's not really colic that's making them miserable — not every issue will go away with time, but genuine colic will).

23

CONSTIPATION
IN BABIES

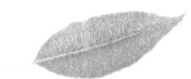

There is nothing more upsetting for a parent than seeing their child unwell. Childhood illnesses have a tendency to be quite intense and distressing. When children get sick, the condition can quickly become severe. With symptoms like bright red rashes, raging fevers, projectile vomiting, or respiratory distress, emergency room visits are not uncommon. But then, as quickly as the condition arrives, it usually resolves itself, leaving the child happily going about her usual activities, with no awareness of the recent gray hairs that have sprouted on her parents' heads.

A child's body has an unencumbered purity that is not found in adults. They are not bogged down by years of heavy food consumption or emotional constraint. They are like an empty vessel, and are much more susceptible to influence from the external environment. This is also why children can heal so completely.

A child's digestive system is very delicate and easily upset. Because they are growing so quickly, they are processing huge amounts of food, which often causes digestive overload. Whereas adults often suffer from indigestion and other ailments because of stress and tension, the opposite is true in children. When there is digestive upset, this can provoke emotional outbursts.

The mother of an eighteen-month-old patient of mine told me that when her child became constipated, his whole personality changed. He went from being a sweet, happy child to a grumpy and difficult one. While a child's emotions are usually uninhibited, buildup in the body can make him feel constrained and physically stagnant. This may cause him to lash out in order to release the feeling of pent-up energy. As children approach the realm of puberty, the tables turn, and constrained emotions become one of the primary causes of illness.

A couple of years ago, I received a call from a mother: her six-month-old infant was crying constantly and not gaining weight. Her doctor recommended that she discontinue nursing and prescribed a formula that she soon realized might not be kosher. The family's rabbi strongly encouraged her to try anything else; he recommended acupuncture. Since she had no prior exposure to acupuncture, she asked me if she could bring her rabbi along.

When they arrived, I took a history and discovered that the child was very constipated. I assessed that the reason he was not gaining weight was because his intestines were totally blocked and not absorbing anything. This is a very common problem in infants. Since he was an otherwise strong child, the prognosis was good. I explained to them that I would use acupuncture to get the intestines moving.

The rabbi then asked, "Why would this be more effective than a laxative?" This was an excellent question. The answer is manifold. Laxatives (even those of herbal origin) bulk or soften the stool, or they act as an irritant to the intestines to stimulate movement. The blockage occurred because the intestines were stalled and needed a boost.

The acupuncture would stimulate movement, which is the same goal as irritant laxatives, except for a major difference: Laxatives can cause dependence and weaken long-term intestinal function, while the acupuncture would stimulate physiologic and automatic intestinal movement and restart independent bowel function.

I warned the mother that since the intestines were so clogged, the acupuncture would probably instigate *a lot* of messy diapers. And that is exactly what happened. Once that cleared up, the baby's intestinal function reverted to normal. He soon began to gain weight happily and healthfully. Thankfully, the mother opted not to listen to her doctor, and continued to nurse. This is (almost always) the best thing for a baby.

Children are a pleasure to treat. Because of their purity, they react very quickly to treatment. Seeing instantaneous results can be very gratifying.

24

BEDWETTING

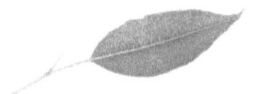

It is widely believed that bedwetting is due to lack of bladder control. While this may be true for some children, for many children the real reason is lack of bladder *capacity*. Often, the bladder's volume is restricted by the contents of the intestines. Bowel buildup is often the cause of bedwetting even in children who don't appear constipated. Many children have regular bowel movements despite serious intestinal accumulation. This is possible because the stool can bypass the intestinal buildup. Daytime or nighttime incontinence is frequently caused by excessive external pressure on the bladder.

In many cases, the bowel buildup is completely symptomless — the only proof that it's there is bedwetting or frequent daytime accidents. Even if there is obvious constipation, most parents and even doctors are unaware of the connection between the bowels and wetting. Most children who are cleared of hidden constipation will experience a complete resolution in bedwetting.

Bowel buildup can also have a systemically harmful effect. It is the hidden cause of urinary tract infections in children (and adults), and is the source of most toilet-training difficulties (whether there is bladder or bowel incontinence, or both). Also, many children with hyperactivity and ADHD can benefit from a bowel cleanse. You may notice bad breath in children with constipation. In fact, most people with bad breath would do well to receive a bowel cleanse. Children with sporadic constipation may have a Jekyll and Hyde sort of temperament: miserable, angry, or out of control when they're constipated, but serene and happy when their bowels are clear. If your child suffers from both mood problems and incontinence, the source is likely a poorly functioning bowel.

In many people, constipation causes intractable headaches. This is mainly because the contents of the bowels are the body's rejects — indigestible, nutritionally worthless or harmful food residue. If this stuff sits around too long, it can release toxins into the bloodstream instead of being eliminated. These toxins can have a detrimental effect on all organ systems, but especially the brain. So what can you do? Use natural methods, such as diet, acupuncture, and exercise and free up constipation.

Some home remedies for constipation:

- Very ripe fruit or dried fruit — especially prunes and figs
- Syrup of figs
- High doses of vitamin C (1000–5000 mg or more)[97]
- Magnesium citrate, which is often in powder form and can be dissolved into drinks
- Chia seeds mixed with water or another liquid

For some children, diminished bladder control may result from some kind of neurological disconnect. Sometimes the problem is due to a weakness of the bladder, which is associated with something Chinese medicine refers to as kidney weakness. Whether the source of the problem is constipation, bladder weakness, or neurological, many children benefit greatly from acupuncture, which can have the effect of rewiring the brain and body.

Sometimes bedwetting has an emotional source, such as anxiety, unhappiness, or trauma. A warning light should go on if you notice a child

---

97 Warning: Do not take over 2000 mg of vitamin C a day during pregnancy; it can cause uterine bleeding and even possibly miscarriage.

who has always been dry suddenly starting to bed-wet, seemingly out of nowhere. Look for changes in mood or possible sources of tension during daytime hours. Some emotional triggers for bedwetting include: being a victim of bullying, homesickness, emotional or physical abuse, or some other kind of shock or trauma. Sometimes even a seemingly small trauma can trigger a strong physical response.

I once made a deal with my daughter when she was four years old that if she stopped using her pacifier, then after three weeks we would get her ears pierced. She agreed to the bargain, and slept like an angel for three weeks, sans pacifier. Then I took her, just the two of us, for a special afternoon of ice cream and ear piercing. That night she held out her hand and asked me, "Can I have my pacie back now?" She had totally misunderstood our deal! I tried to explain it to her, but she went to sleep that night with a broken heart... Then the wetting started.

Riddled with guilt, I gave her back the pacifier, but apparently there was no turning back the clock, as her broken heart (and bladder) persisted. So we put the pacifier away again. Despite the emotional source of her wetting, a few years later, my daughter actually benefited greatly from bowel cleansing. So sometimes the root cause can be multifaceted. Keep in mind that children under six may not have bladder control at night, but many argue that this is a normal phenomenon.

If the source is emotional, it must be addressed, but it is beyond the scope of this book.

25

HEADACHES

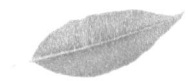

I recently saw an article in a local paper that reported that about one in five children (20 percent) experience headaches. The article went on to explain that parents should not assume the worst, since in most cases there is no serious illness at the root. They advised that brain scans were not usually necessary, and that headaches are nothing to worry about. What the article lacked was the obvious question: Why are so many children suffering? And is there anything that can be done about it?

While headaches in children may be common today, they are certainly not normal. While it is not uncommon for adults to suffer from headaches or migraines, there has been an unprecedented rise in this problem in young children. Another surprise is the increase in seizure disorders. Epilepsy is usually kept confidential by parents, so many are not aware of how common it is.

There are a number of possibly avoidable environmental factors that can trigger seizures and other neurological problems:

- One culprit that is responsible for many headaches, seizures, tics, and other neurological disorders (including Alzheimer's, multiple sclerosis, Parkinson's disease, and many others) is

food additives, especially artificial flavors. The ubiquitous monosodium glutamate (MSG) and aspartame are the biggest culprits.

- Another insidious trigger for neurological problems is **heavy metals**, like mercury, aluminum, and lead. Watch out for silver (amalgam) dental fillings, which are comprised of 50 percent mercury, as well as medications containing thimerosal. Also be careful not to allow aluminum to come into direct contact with food.

MSG is a food additive that is notorious for causing headaches, in addition to triggering ADHD and other acute and chronic neurological problems. If you have headaches (actually, if you have a pulse!) eliminate all MSG from your diet. Beware of MSG hidden on food labels under lesser-known names like autolyzed yeast extract, hydrolyzed vegetable or soy protein, and even "natural flavors"!

Artificial sweeteners commonly found in sodas and chewing gum and other "sugar-free" sweet foods have a similarly disastrous effect, causing headaches and other neurological problems. Artificial flavors, colors, and preservatives (like sulfites and nitrates) are another common headache trigger. So, in essence, it is best to avoid all food additives. Beware that dried fruit and most wine and grape juice contain preservatives, which can be a headache trigger.

Any child or adult who experiences headaches or another neurological problem should stay far from all food additives. If removing the above additives does not bring about complete headache resolution, consider removing gluten, a sensitivity that affects a smaller minority of people. Another less common trigger is soy, which can be hidden in bakery products, but is otherwise usually found on food labels.

Other common causes of headaches include:

- Withdrawal from medications — most commonly from psychiatric drugs such as stimulants, but even nonprescription drugs (like Benadryl) may be the culprit.

- Dehydration — this sort of headache does not usually occur on a daily basis, unlike those that are the result of exposure to one of the triggers mentioned above. Offer drinks (naturally flavored) to children complaining of headaches to rule out dehydration.
- Exhaustion or lack of sleep — this type of headache is more common in adults, who generally deprive themselves of sleep more regularly than do children.
- Stress-induced headaches — these are more common in adults, but may arise in teens as well. Sometimes this can be related to jaw clenching and teeth grinding.
- Constipation — this is a lesser-known cause of headaches. In these cases, the headache will resolve itself when the constipation is cleared.

Many parents tell me that removing the artificial junk foods from their children's diets will be too difficult. I usually share the following analogy: If a child had a deadly peanut allergy, there would be no question about strict adherence to a peanut-free diet. Both the parent and the school will do everything in their power to keep the child away from the offending nut.

Sensitivities to additives like MSG are very common. Though the reaction may not be as immediate or severe as anaphylaxis, unbeknown to many, these additives can cause devastating physical, cognitive, and neurological problems in both children and adults. There is good reason to treat MSG sensitivity as seriously as you would a peanut allergy. A child who is old enough to understand its effects will usually cooperate fully. Include him on shopping trips and have him read food labels to get him involved in improving and taking responsibility for his own health.

26

ASTHMA

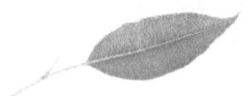

The incidence of asthma is on the rise. It is a frightening and danger-ous disease. Modern medicine labels most cases of asthma as chronic and incurable.

I have witnessed the following situation numerous times:

> *A child catches a cold, which turns into a severe cough. He may develop a fever as the cough transforms into bronchitis. A visit to the doctor and a prescription for antibiotics brings the fever down. For some reason, once the course of antibiotics is complete, the child is still coughing. This cycle repeats itself for months... Then, due to some trigger (dietary, emotional, environmental), the child suddenly experiences a frightening wheeze or shortness of breath.*
>
> *Another trip to the doctor leads to a diagnosis of asthma and prescriptions for bronchodilators, steroids, or other antiasthmatics. The mother, who has watched the con-dition progress through every stage, may say to herself,*

*"Hey, this isn't asthma! I remember when this all start-
ed — it was that cold. Before that, my child never had
any breathing issues. Now he has to depend on inhalers
for the rest of his life?"*

While the above scenario is not the only way asthma can develop, it is a very common route, and very treatable with natural medicine. There is no reason for a cough to linger for months on end, opening the way for chronic breathing disturbance. At any point, even after a diagnosis of asthma, this process can be reversed, leading the child to a healthy state once again. Don't wait for a diagnosis of asthma to seek out alternatives to the typical treatments with antibiotics or steroids.

Asthma that was not a direct result of a lung infection, but seems to have developed on its own, may be a sign of a more severe deficiency in the body. One may observe that this type of child (or adult) often seems weak or tired, with low resistance to illness. In these cases, the internal environment is paramount. While it can take time to strengthen an individual whose reserves are low, these people are still treatable, even curable.

Asthma is usually considered to be an allergic disorder whose management mainly entails identifying and then avoiding the specific allergens that act as triggers. From a holistic perspective, triggers such as dust mites, pollen, or mold are merely the final straw. Individuals will put a lot of effort and money into eliminating these triggers. While it is sensible to improve one's environment, the true problem is *within* the body, and that is where most of the effort should be aimed.

Bronchodilators can be lifesaving in emergency situations. Furthermore, once an individual has become dependent on inhalers, they become indispensable (for the time being). However, prolonged use may lead to addiction even in small children. Worse still, while they expand the airways in the short term, over time they weaken the lungs and can exacerbate the severity of the asthma.

In breathing dysfunction, there is often a buildup of stubborn mucus in the lungs. While conventional drugs dilate the bronchi and make breathing easier, in addition to weakening the lungs they do not clear out the substances that are clogging the bronchi.

As far as holistic medicine is concerned, asthma is curable. Long-term use of addictive antiasthmatic drugs makes the condition more stubborn, but not impossible to treat. The goals of treatment are to clear accumulated mucus and to strengthen the lung deficiency. The results are very good. With the ultimate goal being to cure the asthma, it is well worth the effort.

The following are some tips for asthma treatment:

1. Since most cases of asthma involve chronic phlegm, individuals should avoid phlegm-producing foods, like dairy, peanuts, sugar, and possibly wheat. Removing one food at a time for at least three weeks to test for improvement may be easier than eliminating all possible triggers at once.

2. If a child (aged five years or older) is hyperventilating, have them breathe into a paper bag. During hyperventilation, the lungs become over-oxygenated, and the recycled CO_2 will calm and slow the breathing.

3. Blow up a balloon ten times every day. Practiced preventatively, this will strengthen the lungs and increase lung capacity. This exercise has been shown to be as effective in the treatment of asthma as bronchodilators, but without weakening the lungs. (Caution: balloons are a common choking hazard; do not leave them lying around in homes with small children.)

4. If the child has a dry cough, or very dry lips, turn on a steamy shower to create a warm humidifier. Note that humidifiers are only beneficial to children suffering from dry conditions and may not be beneficial to a child with a wet, gurgling cough (see tip #1). With a dry cough, there may be mucus as well, but that mucus will be of the thick, gluey, dry variety.

Final notes: Before vaccination became widespread, it was common knowledge that "no child dies from asthma." Nobody would make this statement about asthma today. Sadly, with the advent of certain vaccines (DPT probably being the first), rates of asthma have increased manifold, and it has become epidemic and far more deadly. Vaccination is continuously causing many new cases of asthma, and has turned it into a common and deadly disease — so buyer beware.

27

ALLERGIES

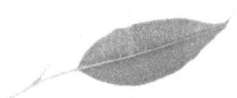

My husband's grandfather used to say, "What's with all these 'allergies'? In my day, there were people who were sensitive to wool...or leather...but nothing like today."

Half a century ago, food allergies were virtually unheard of. Occasionally you'd find someone with sensitivities to certain foods (such as strawberries), but it was a rarity.

If there was one child in a class who was allergic to something, it was a conversation piece.

Some might scoff at this *zeidy* (grandpa) and say that he was just ignorant. That in his day nobody knew how to diagnose things like allergies, but since then, science and education have advanced, so we are picking up on problems that used to be mysterious and nameless. I would tend to disagree. If the problem existed in those days, people would have picked up on it. In reality, I believe that it is not the diagnostics that are cutting edge, but the diseases. (Yes, many diagnostic tests are new, but they were created to accommodate the changing health profile of society — they are a *reflection* of the change, not the *source* of our awareness.)

170

Today, allergies have become the rule, not the exception. What has changed in recent years that has so dramatically altered our reaction to food?

Furthermore, food allergies do not occur equally throughout the world. They are far less common in less-modernized countries, especially those with little Western medical care. In the US, food allergies have doubled during the past ten years alone. What has changed during this time?[98]

OBVIOUS CHANGES

During the last few decades, society has become increasingly interested in health foods. What has led to this new fad? The truth is that the need for health food stems from the unhealthy direction that the current food market has taken. Traditionally, crops were unadulterated and free of harmful chemicals and synthetic, factory-made ingredients. There was no need for a separate section in the supermarket. Today, genetically modified, processed, packaged, nutritionally-stripped foods make up the bulk of our diet. In contrast, go back a few generations, and you will find that all that was available was locally grown, fresh organic produce.

Cows were not fed corn, nor their dead, diseased counterparts (cows grazed and ate their natural diet of grass, shrubs, leaves, etc.). Neither were they subjected to hormones and antibiotics like they are today. Tomatoes were not altered with fish DNA so that they can survive frigid weather. Not so long ago, toxic pesticides and chemical fertilizers were unheard of.

Traditionally, wheat was the staple grain in many societies. Today, however, it has become the culprit for many ailments, from wheat allergies to celiac disease (a debilitating autoimmune condition where the body cannot tolerate gluten). In light of wheat bread's historic role as the essential dietary element, why are so many allergic to it today?

It is precisely because of wheat's popularity that is has become allergenic. There are few crops in the world that have been altered as

---

98   Heather Fraser, *The Peanut Allergy Epidemic*, 2011.

much as wheat to improve productivity and profitability. It has been genetically modified to survive extreme temperature changes. It has also been modified to greatly increase the amount of gluten it contains (see celiac disease above). The wheat we eat today is so far removed from its origins, it's no wonder it is making so many people sick!

INSIDIOUS CHANGES

Aside from the nature of food, it appears that the nature of the human body has changed as well. Allergies are explained as a misdirected immune response, where the food is being treated as a foreign disease-causing agent, and the body reacts to it in much the same way that it would to a foreign microorganism.

What has caused our immune system to react to food as if it were a disease?

Now that we understand the possibility of strange genetic material (as well as chemicals and additives being part of most foods today), immune response to food makes sense: our bodies don't like the food we are ingesting.

There is another possibility as well.

Around 1913, experiments were conducted where casein (a milk protein) or egg lecithin were emulsified with various vegetable oils (corn, cottonseed, castor, and more). When injected, these various formulations were known to induce anaphylaxis (a potentially deadly allergic response) and also to trigger future sensitivity to these products.

The vitamin K shot given at birth contains castor seed oil (a legume similar to peanut) and the hepatitis B shot contains casein (from milk). Soy allergies began appearing in infants at three months, which was the age that babies began receiving the pneumococcal vaccine, which contains soy peptone. The MMR (measles, mumps, rubella) vaccine contained chick embryo, and sparked an ever-rising trend in egg allergies.[99]

The above food items are not the only victims. Barbara Feick Gregory, a vaccine researcher, was surprised to discover that for nearly every

---

99   Ibid.

food allergy that exists today, "that food was listed as an ingredient in a vaccine adjuvant or culture medium." The incidence of allergies in vaccinated children is more than double that of unvaccinated.

So why might food in vaccines cause allergies? Vaccines are injected with the intention of causing an immune response. Aside from the disease entity, other (non-health promoting) substances are added to increase the body's immune response; because of this, the body may recognize other ingredients in the injection, not only the disease, as an antigen (a foreign substance that the body must fight). This can reprogram the immune system to indefinitely respond to certain foods as if they were diseases.

After penicillin was introduced, there was a strange phenomenon where many people developed often fatal anaphylaxis and dangerous allergic responses to ingredients in the medication. What most people are not aware of is *why* penicillin triggered this reaction: in order to boost potency, penicillin was given via injection rather than orally. Further, **peanut oil** was added to the penicillin injections to slow absorption of the drug and make a dose last longer in the body. If penicillin had only been given orally, allergic or anaphylactic reactions to the drug would probably never have occurred.

Anything taken by mouth will be processed through the digestive system, allowing only certain components to reach the bloodstream. Injection bypasses the body's digestive infrastructure and introduces foreign proteins directly into the bloodstream. When the body recognizes these allergenic proteins as foreign, it is not due to an immunological malfunction at all. It is a predictable immune response to a foreign substance (antigen) that has been unnaturally and forcibly introduced to the bloodstream, where it does not belong. It is not specifically vaccination or antibiotics that cause allergies or anaphylaxis, it is the hypodermic needle and the *injection* of foreign proteins directly into the bloodstream that triggers a predictable but unwanted immune response.

Since allergies are a learned or programmed immune response to specific antigenic components in certain foods, they can be very difficult to reverse. I will, however, give a few tips to help mitigate or possibly even eliminate allergies. At the very least, some of these tips may help you to detect sensitivities.

- If you discover that you are allergic to a certain food, even if the allergy creates subtler symptoms like stomach discomfort or lethargy, try eliminating the trigger food from your diet for at least a year. During this time, your body may actually heal as gut inflammation improves, and the immune reaction may completely vanish. Therefore, if the reaction was never life-threatening, but more of a mild discomfort, you can attempt to slowly and cautiously reintroduce the food while observing for reactions (if you miss the food terribly).
- Consider trying a GAPS diet, which includes a lot of healing bone broths and natural food-based probiotics. This must be done in the absence of trigger foods.[100]
- Test your reaction to more whole versions of the trigger foods; i.e., if you have a problem with wheat, you may still find that organic sprouted wheat does not give you trouble, or that grass-fed unhomogenized dairy is better than the conventional products. You can try these foods at the beginning of an elimination diet. If you see no improvement in allergy symptoms, avoid the more natural versions of trigger foods as well.
- To test for an allergic response, you can try swiping the food (wet) on your wrist and leaving it overnight. If there is redness in the area, you are having an inflammatory reaction to that food.

I do know people who have meticulously avoided trigger foods for one year or more and were eventually able to reintroduce foods into their diets without experiencing allergic reactions; however, there are no guarantees.

---

100   Natasha Campbell McBride, MD, Gut and Psychology Syndrome: *Natural Treatment for Autism, ADD/ADHD, Dyslexia, Dyspraxia*, 2004.

Leaky gut syndrome is known as a state in which the intestines are inflamed and therefore allowing improperly digested food or waste products to pass unhindered into the bloodstream, resulting in inflammation in other bodily systems as well.

Although leaky gut is a hypothetical construct (as far as I can tell), the concept of a gut disorder causing widespread systemic havoc in the body is well recognized in Chinese medicine. This is particularly true in pediatrics, where some say that most conditions are rooted in the (lack of) health of the digestive tract. This is something that I have seen in action many times.

SIMPLE BONE BROTH RECIPE

- Buy chicken necks or feet, turkey necks, or other poultry or cow bones, including marrow bones. (Alternatively, fish bones may be used.) Use any combination of animal bones — the more the better.
- Place the bones in a large pot and add enough water to cover the bones generously.
- Add a tablespoon of apple cider vinegar (which will leach the minerals out of the bones).
- Some let the combination sit for one hour (I don't).
- Bring to a boil, then lower to a simmer, checking intermittently and adding water as needed. Cook covered.
- Optional: skim the foam off the top. (I don't bother with this, since I filter all the scum out at the end anyway, using a large mesh spoon.)

- Simmer on low for twenty-four to seventy-two hours. (Again, these are the official instructions — I often cook bone broth for less than twenty-four hours when I have a time constraint or deadline. The cooking time is flexible.)
- Remove the bones and add salt and pepper to taste. (Don't be stingy with the salt, just use a good, healthy, unrefined salt.)
- Vegetables — some recipes advise adding the vegetables before the long cooking stretch and then discarding everything except the liquid. I think that this is unnecessary and wasteful. Instead, I recommend that after the one-to-three-day bone-cooking period, remove the bones and then add your choice of vegetable and cook to your liking (about two to six hours).
- Suggested vegetable ideas (use any combination): carrots, zucchini, butternut squash, onions (chopped or whole), kohlrabi, parsnip, celery (root, leaves, or stalks), parsley, dill, and more.

SEASONAL ALLERGIES

Allergies come in two very different forms. We discussed food allergies above, but seasonal allergies or hay fever are also widespread. Some common symptoms include itchy, sore, or red eyes, sneezing, runny or stuffed nose, and exhaustion. Many view this as an overzealous immune reaction, where the body recognizes safe substances (i.e., pollen, dander, hay...) as foreign.

Antihistamines are often prescribed in order to dull the body's overreaction. While these drugs often help reduce allergy symptoms, they have no effect on the long-term condition, and individuals will continue to suffer year after year. In other words, antihistamines can only provide temporary symptom relief. There is also a major flaw in the objective of this medication, which will help us understand why it is incapable of bringing about a cure.

The patients I see who suffer from seasonal allergies do not appear to have strong immune systems at all. In fact, their defenses are so low that these individuals are often the sorts who catch every bug that comes their way. From a holistic perspective, it is a weakness in the body's defenses that truly causes these people to suffer through allergy season. Suppressing the immune system is really quite counterproductive if one has any hope of ridding themselves of their allergies.

So why do these individuals suffer more in the spring (or fall)? The change of seasons is when our defenses must work their hardest, since our temperature regulatory system must acclimate to sudden environmental changes. Those of us who suffer most are those whose bodies have some trouble adjusting to climate changes quickly.

So although on a molecular level, allergy sufferers may seem to be overreacting to pollen, etc., in truth, they usually have an extremely weak immune system. The ultimate proof of this is that these individuals get better with treatments that strengthen their immune system. If this was really a pure overreaction, then strengthening the immunity should cause their allergies to get worse (which does not happen).

When an individual comes to me at the peak of allergy season, the goal of treatment is to allay their symptoms. We do so in much the same way that we would when treating someone who is suffering from a cold or flu. However, the goal is never to suppress the immune reaction. Rather, we *strengthen* the immune system so that it is able to eliminate pathogens.

This works much better for colds than it does for chronic allergies. This is because when patients are suffering from an acute attack of a chronic condition, we must treat the acute symptoms before we can address the underlying condition. Every condition has layers. In order to treat the innermost layers and bring about a cure, you must first eliminate the external layers, i.e., the acute symptoms; only then can you deal with the underlying systemic imbalance.

28

PARASITES

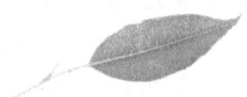

Parasites are widespread, and they cause problems in all age groups. Chronic recurrent parasitic infections can be rather stubborn and very difficult to eliminate. For people with chronic parasitic infection, eliminating parasites can be a long, difficult, and frustrating process, but don't give up — it's worth the effort.

I have heard people say, "Only people in third-world countries suffer from parasitic infection." This is erroneous. Parasites are quite common in affluent countries as well, though there is certainly a higher distribution of parasitic infections in warmer climates.

In small children, hygiene and bad habits are obvious contributing factors. Some children are always putting things in their mouths, or sucking their fingers, thereby potentially reintroducing parasitic worms. Parasites can be harbored under fingernails. Therefore, make sure to keep children's nails very short, and ensure that they clean their hands after using the bathroom.

Not everyone who suffers from parasites contracts them through thumb-sucking. Parasites can be harbored in food and water supplies as well (melons and cucumbers are often blamed). They can come from animal feces, and may be found in soil or sandboxes. Many people with chronic infection are not reintroducing parasites through ingestion. The worms are living inside them all the time. Sometimes they are dormant, and sometimes active, but they can be ever-present.

A number of years ago, a woman in her thirties came to me for treatment for chronic parasites that she had been suffering from since she was a small child! She reported that Vermox seemed to have no effect on the situation. She told me that her doctor offended her by giving her a lecture about hygiene, "Does he think I don't wash my hands?" In her case, as with most adults, the presence of parasites had nothing to do with personal hygiene.

What causes parasites to become chronic in some individuals to the point where the worms are impervious to antiparasitic drugs? One possibility is buildup in the intestines, creating blockages that allow the worms to find places to set up permanent residence. Vermox is often ineffective when the intestines are clogged — the parasites can hide from the drug and continue to thrive.

If intestines are working well, then even if one ingests parasites they should pass right through, because they have nowhere to settle. Therefore, one of the main goals of treatment is to eliminate blockages and create healthy intestinal movement. Aside from healthy movement without buildup, another factor is a healthy intestinal environment, which is the result of eating right. The main foods to avoid are sugar and white flour, or any "fast carbs." If parasites are found to be an issue, even fruit should be kept to a minimum.

Parasitic worm infections are far more common than we realize. Only a small percentage of the millions of people harboring parasites are even aware of the condition. There may be no symptoms, or there may be abdominal pain, insomnia, nausea, weight loss, and increased or decreased appetite.

The most common parasitic culprit in affluent countries is pinworm, the smallest worm in the helminth family. Symptoms include itching or stinging in the anal or perineal area at night, and possibly insomnia, restlessness, emotional instability, and loss of appetite and bladder control. Sometimes a child is diagnosed with ADHD when in fact, their behavioral problems are due to chronic worm infection. It may be worth treating an emotionally labile child for worms just in case that is the source of their suffering.

There are numerous dietary changes that can be helpful in eliminating worms:

1. Food should be **chewed** thoroughly to promote better digestion.
2. Parasites thrive on **sugar**. Aside from avoiding junk food, you will starve worms by avoiding sweet fruits. **Parasites do not like sour foods**, so berries, pomegranate, lemon, (and possibly grapefruit) can be eaten.
3. Antiparasitic foods include the following raw vegetables: beet, cabbage, carrot, onion, radish, and **garlic**, washed well and peeled. (Only children with strong digestion can tolerate a lot of raw vegetables.) Take at least one clove of garlic daily. Lightly roasted **pumpkin seeds** destroy parasites, and a handful can be snacked on daily. Eat garlic and pumpkin seeds between meals to enhance their potency. **Papaya** has antiparasitic properties, so it is also highly recommended.

    I used to give the following advice, which I extracted from a book in my health library: "Garlic can be made more tolerable to children by slicing thinly and placing between slices of green apple." Then, one day, it occurred to me that this was ridiculous advice! From a culinary perspective, garlic and apples are an unpalatable combination. Instead, you can try chopping or crushing garlic cloves and putting them in salads, dips, or spreads where they belong and actually taste great! Food does not have to taste terrible or bizarre to be medicinal.

4. **Mugwort** is a mild herb that encourages the elimination of parasites and improves digestive function. Drink one cup of mugwort tea two hours after dinner. Caution: some herbal traditions believe that this herb is contraindicated (forbidden) during pregnancy.

5. Some more powerful herbs to treat parasites include **black walnut, cloves, and wormwood**. The three together can make a potent combination. There are various methods for using these herbs, so it is best to read up on the best way to use these herbs for your family.

6. **Probiotics**: Healthy intestinal flora (bacteria) can help combat harmful foreign organisms. While there are many strains on the market, lactobacillus acidophilus is one of the few that has been proven safe and effective. Live yogurt is also a probiotic; buy only *unsweetened*. A few teaspoons daily are all that is needed to reestablish intestinal flora. Raw sauerkraut also contains beneficial bacteria.

7. There is evidence that making the body more **alkaline** (as opposed to acidic) through dietary changes can help eliminate parasites, because parasites thrive in a more acidic intestinal environment.

THE pH DIET

There is much debate in the area of eating to alkalize the body, and I believe that there are many unproven claims. The basis upon which many foods are being categorized as alkalizing and therefore health-promoting, or acidifying and therefore unhealthy, still stands on shaky ground. Alkaline diet advocates forbid many foods that are potentially health-promoting according to other effective systems, which is why I take the pH advice with a grain of salt. Also, although people who are ill tend to run at a lower pH (i.e., more acidic), it is difficult to prove which comes first: Does an acidic environment cause disease? Or does disease or poor health cause the body to become more acidic?

Since this is relatively uncharted territory, time will tell us what's really going on. In the interim, assuming that the pH theory is correct (and it seems plausible that some of these nutritional measures have the potential to improve health), and that the foods that are presumed to alkalize the body in fact do so, one may try some of the following health tips toward that end:

- Eat nutrient-dense vegetables and fruit including seaweeds and blue-green algae. (This is general pH advice; for worm infection, limit intake of sweet fruit.)
- Use herbs like parsley, basil, dill, and cilantro.
- Prepare bone broth that contains many alkaline minerals, as well as amino acids (protein). See the chapter on allergies for a simple bone broth recipe.
- For a short time period (about three days), one can try taking fresh vegetable juice and bone broth exclusively.
- Drink quality mineral water (which is free of fluoride), even adding a pinch of salt or baking soda.
- Use unrefined salts with high mineral content, such as gray volcanic salts, pink Himalayan salt, or unrefined, unprocessed ocean salt. Refined sea salt should be avoided.

8. **Spice it up**: Parasites do not like hot, spicy foods. Eat cayenne pepper as an antiparasitic remedy.
9. **Citrus seeds** have antiparasitic qualities. Some people purchase citrus seed extract. You can also collect lemon and grapefruit

seeds, grind them up and mix them with honey. The honey attracts the worms and the citrus seeds will (hopefully) kill them.

10. **Pray**. Worms are stubborn. You need all the help you can get!

Some people need intestinal-cleansing treatments that are more powerful than a home remedy can provide. Also, many antiparasitic herbs cannot be self-prescribed. An herbal practitioner should be sought out for stubborn or complex cases.

29

ACNE

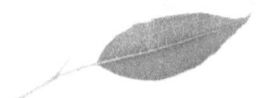

Acne is a poorly timed condition. Teenagers, for whom appearance is paramount, make up the majority of acne sufferers. Some like to blame everything on hormones, even if no imbalance is detectable. Hormones often serve as the culprit when the true cause of the condition is unknown.

PHARMACEUTICALS

Doctors may prescribe powerful antibiotics, such as tetracycline, for long-term treatment of acne. Antibiotics are not very successful in eliminating the condition and cause many harmful side effects, making them a poor treatment choice.

During the past few decades, the prescription drug Accutane made quite a name for itself, since it effectively cures many cases of acne. Then, after close to thirty years on the market, its manufacturers stopped producing the drug. It seems they were losing too much money in lawsuits implicating the drug for causing inflammatory bowel disease. The medication was also known for causing miscarriages and birth defects, as well as depression and even suicide.

Side effects can get rather strange while taking this drug. A patient of mine reported that while taking the medication, when she tried to have her eyebrows waxed her skin would peel off. Another patient reported that years after taking the drug, his skin would darken if he took a hot shower. The drug seems to accumulate in the skin and remain there interminably.

While no other drug has ever come close to Accutane in effectiveness, with all the possible dangers, it is questionable whether this drug is worth the risk. There are still generic versions of this medication available, but there is no reason to believe that they are any less risky than the original. This is a drug to **especially avoid during reproductive years**. I only hope that patients are adequately warned of its potential to cause birth defects by prescribing physicians.

DIET

When I was a child, I remember seeing a "science" program on PBS that talked about acne. They stated definitively that chocolate has no effect on acne. Though I was probably still in elementary school, and did not have too many peers suffering from the condition, I knew that what they were saying was wrong. Everybody knows that chocolate can trigger acne in *certain* individuals. Many acne sufferers can report decisively which foods trigger their acne.

DIETARY RECOMMENDATIONS

Though diet alone may not be enough to cure every case, it is often paramount in the treatment of acne. Stay away from greasy and spicy foods. Avoid white carbs, sugar, dairy, citrus fruits, and red meat. Acne sufferers usually do well with small amounts of unrefined sesame oil. Most benefit from a diet high in fresh vegetables, especially carrots, pumpkin, and winter squash, leafy greens, and unpeeled (but thoroughly washed) cucumbers. Seaweed is also very therapeutic.

Acne can come in many different forms. In practice, we make the diagnosis by looking at the location of the acne, the color, presence of oil or dryness, and, of course, the overall constitution of the patient. Acne sufferers usually have a lot of heat in their systems. This can be seen in the redness and inflammation found in the condition. The redder the acne or overall complexion, the more heat present in the individual. This is the reason it is important to avoid spicy, warming foods.

From a Chinese medical perspective, Accutane and antibiotics are extremely cold in nature, and eliminate a tremendous amount of heat from the system. However, their side effects make them a dangerous choice. I prefer to prescribe herbal remedies that can be cooling and balancing, addressing the underlying condition without inflicting undue damage.

SELF-HELP

- Aloe vera gel can be applied generously over the areas affected by acne. It has anti-inflammatory and antibacterial properties. It can also help heal and regenerate the skin.
- Fresh lemon juice has antiseptic qualities. Dab directly onto the lesions, or mix one teaspoon lemon juice with one tablespoon water and use as a face wash twice daily. (Be careful not to get lemon in your eyes.)
- Tea tree essential oil is a powerful antiseptic. Apply one drop to pus-filled lesions twice daily. Discontinue if severe irritation occurs. It is recommended not to ingest essential oil. (See home remedies section for more information.)
- Nutritional supplements: vitamins A (do not overdose!), B complex, and C, as well as zinc, and omega-3 essential oils are helpful.

30

ADHD

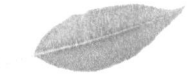

During the past few decades, many parents have been warned by educators or doctors that children with "undiagnosed" or unmedicated ADHD are likely to become "kids at risk," and eventually end up on the street as criminals and drug addicts. It makes one wonder: Are they suggesting that the way to *prevent* drug addiction is by *giving* children drugs? Administering drugs to prevent drug addiction is done under the pretext that there is a major difference between psychoactive prescription drugs and nonprescription illegal narcotics. But is there?

Today, it is in vogue for principals and teachers to act as psychiatric diagnosticians (or at least referral agencies for psychiatric evaluation). In addition to claiming extensive knowledge and experience in child psychology, many educators seem to be under the impression that they have uncanny prophetic abilities.

Perhaps there is some sort of annual conference for principals where, among other things, they are taught that children with ADHD who are left untreated (with medication) will become kids at risk. It sure seems that way, because everywhere I turn I am hearing this exact same refrain. Principals of schools across the world are giving parents virtually *the exact same prediction*. Is there a basis for this prediction, and where is it coming from?

Perhaps it is coming from their own experience, as they claim, but I find this doubtful. People are far too unpredictable to manage to create such consistency — that most (or many) untreated children with ADHD should eventually become criminals or drug addicts really does not do justice to human nature, so I reject the notion that personal experience has led to these conclusions. Psychiatric drug expert Dr. Peter Breggin, MD, seems to have found the real source for this popular prediction:

According to Dr. Breggin, since the 1990s,

> Doctors have begun to warn parents that the long-range outcome for children who have ADHD is not good unless they receive treatment. These doctors mention studies showing that boys diagnosed with ADHD will suffer from a higher incidence of criminal behavior and other problems in young adulthood...
>
> But there is a catch to the studies: The children who grew up to have problems were being treated with Ritalin. In fact, the treatment was conducted free, at an advanced 'no-cost clinic.' These reports should discourage parents from handing over their children to the doctors. [The studies] suggest that **being diagnosed with ADHD and being treated with Ritalin leads to a long-term negative outcome.**"[101] [102]

There is a pervasive belief that society today, and particularly the educational system, is somehow more enlightened than it was in the past. While it certainly is *different*, in reality, more children than ever before are being diagnosed with various disorders and receiving intervention at or through their schools. In some cases, this may be a truly wonderful

---

101   Breggin, PR, MD, *Talking Back to Ritalin*, revised edition, 2001.

102   Klein RG, Mannuzza S. "Long-term outcome of hyperactive children: A review," *J Am Acad Child Adolesc Psychiatry*. 1991 May;30(3):383–7.

thing, and may be helping many children develop. On the other hand, the eagerness to label as many children as possible with developmental disorders has the potential to cause harm as well.

Although we are living in the information age, where modern technology, media, and communication are advancing rapidly, society as a whole is deteriorating. The school system is not immune to this trend. In reality, modern schools are very intolerant of children who do not fit into the increasingly narrow definition of normal. How many parents have received the ultimatum, "Drugs or out"? They are made to feel guilty, irresponsible, and even spiritually destructive for their noncompliance to medicate their children. Many parents are terrified by the idea of their child being kicked out of school or becoming an at-risk kid, so they acquiesce and get the prescription filled.

Attention Deficit Hyperactive Disorder is truly the best example of this attempt to cure children of their personalities. Rather than creatively coming up with methods to reach each child individually, whether his problem is sensory, social, learning, behavioral, or other, our schools search relentlessly for diagnoses in order to blame the child (victim) for any problems he is suffering from at school.

PRESCRIPTION-DRUG ADDICTION

What about the predictions that undrugged children with ADHD will become drug addicts (and criminals)? I have received numerous calls from people reporting the exact opposite experience. Children and adults of all ages start psychiatric drugs according to doctor's orders, but frequently become addicted and end up engaging in risky behaviors. For many, their personalities change in the typical fashion of a drug addict. Of course, the victim is then blamed for "abusing" their drugs.

In reality, many people are transformed into drug addicts while using medication as prescribed. Often, when patients report side effects, their psychiatrist will add another drug to their regimen. This drug cocktail frequently leads to further deterioration, which is often blamed on the patient's underlying condition. The effects of most psychiatric-drug combinations have not been properly tested for potential interactions. This makes the patient the experimental subject.

The main reason that people who are taking prescription drugs may be less likely to resort to street drugs (if there is any truth to that assertion) is because easy access to prescription narcotics makes acquiring drugs on the street wholly unnecessary. Nevertheless, these people are not being *saved* from a life of drug addiction, just the *inconvenience* of acquiring them illegally.

DON'T COMPARE

Many parents become disheartened when they compare their own child to other people's kids. Or worse yet, when *educators* compare their child's performance to others. Just because other children can sit really quietly for a long time doesn't mean that there is something wrong with a child who can't. If one in ten American children is being drugged for hyperactivity, then we can be sure that it's really a normal way to be. Many of these children are bursting with energy and enthusiasm, which may get them far one day.

One of the reasons that some children don't respond to anything besides drugs is because there may be nothing wrong with them in the first place. Being bored and restless in school is hardly a mental illness! How much pleasure would adults get and how much patience would they have if they were forced to sit and listen to the same lecturers all day long, day after day? Yet this is what is required of all children, and when they have trouble staying focused and become restless in school, the conclusion is that there must be something wrong with the child.

One principal derisively proclaimed to parents of a restless boy, "In a previous generation, your son would have been sent to work on a farm!" And then elaborated that in today's educational model, less scholarly or more energetic children have the "privilege" of being fixed (with drugs) and mainstreamed.

Is there anything wrong with farming? Is there only one path of learning and development that works for all children? For the most part, adults have the luxury of choosing a career path that suits their skills and personalities. Children don't have a choice.

If your school is demanding that your child be diagnosed with and medicated for ADHD or any other psychiatric disorder, ask yourself — and them — the following questions:

- Are these drugs free of serious risks?
- What are common side effects of the drugs being offered?
- What effect will they have on my child's growth, overall health, and happiness?
- What effect will stimulants have on my child's brain development, learning, memory, and personality?
- Are they addictive? What are common withdrawal symptoms, and how will they affect my child's life?
- Will my child be able to go off these drugs easily?
- If he goes off the drugs, will he be in better or worse shape than before he started?
- Who benefits most from stimulants? Will stimulants be good for my child in the long run?
- Are they worth the risk?

Most educators don't ask these questions, nor do they know the answers to them. However, if they don't *want* to know the answers, then perhaps they are not in the best position to advise on such a serious decision.

The arbitrary diagnostic criteria for ADHD have become so broad that almost any adult or child could easily be given this label! Many people cannot fit into the increasingly narrow definition of normal.

As I see it, people who are diagnosed with ADD/ADHD fall into one of two categories:

- A true behavioral/brain imbalance or deficit
- A personality type where the child is just not fitting into the box

How can you tell the difference? One way is to ask yourself some of the following questions:

- If the term and symptom list for ADHD didn't exist, would this person still be seen as abnormal or mentally compromised in any way?

- Would the person have received a diagnosis in the 1950s (or 1850s for that matter)?
- Are the "symptoms" only a problem at school (as opposed to weekends or summer vacation)? Did the problems only appear after starting school?
- Does the person have any physical symptoms or serious learning delays?

As for adults with an ADHD diagnosis, it may seem nice to be able say, "I cannot succeed because I have a disability," but I suspect that this does more harm than good. While some of the tools shared in adult ADHD support groups may be wise and beneficial, are we truly better off when we give our challenges a psychiatric diagnosis? I remain unconvinced.

Rather than empowering people to improve their lives, an ADHD diagnosis may have the opposite effect. The label may give one an excuse to fail or even a *license* to fail! However, life is full of seemingly insurmountable challenges. When we are offered quick and easy solutions to complicated problems, we must stop and think. There are no shortcuts. No matter which path we choose, we are going to have to work to reach our goal. Drugs may seem like the simplest solution. But raising children (and adults) is not easy.

If you find that an ADHD diagnosis helps you reach your goals and accomplish more, then great! But if it is disabling and leaves you feeling like a powerless victim, then you may be better off remembering that it doesn't take very much to receive an ADHD diagnosis. The evidence that the incredibly common traits that lead to an ADHD diagnosis have a basis in a genuine disorder remains shaky.

WHY STIMULANTS WORK "BEST"

One of the reasons for the perception that stimulants "work" when alternative options sometimes don't is because stimulants can "cure" a person of his personality! If nothing is out of balance, no amount of acupuncture, vitamin supplementation, craniosacral therapy, herbal remedies, etc., will succeed in altering one's underlying nature. Drugs, however, will suppress a person's behavior, even if nothing is wrong.

ADHD is diagnosed without regard for the varying talents, strengths, and shortcomings of individuals. Energetic children who cannot "conform" have all the potential for success if given the right tools. Interestingly, there is a large contingent of children diagnosed with ADHD who are actually geniuses, and for whom the modern school system was not designed.

If there is a *true* imbalance, then I recommend first seeking out any and every alternative to drugs. Many holistic treatments are aimed at addressing and treating the underlying problems and can be highly effective in helping improve children's behavior, learning, and even overall health. Chinese medicine, acupuncture, craniosacral therapy, heavy metal detoxification, nutritional supplementation, dietary therapy, vision therapy, various brain exercise programs, and more have all been effective in reducing hyperactivity and improving learning and concentration when a genuine imbalance is present.

31

STIMULANTS

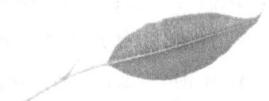

EVADING THE SYSTEM

One woman shared the following story with me:

> *I was very upset when my husband told me that he took Ritalin as a child. But recently my mother-in-law told me a part of the story that was unknown to all involved until now.*

This is her mother-in law's story:

> *During my son's elementary school years, the school administration insisted that we put him on medication for ADHD. We visited a psychiatrist, who was more than happy to diagnose my son with ADHD and prescribe Ritalin. I bought a bottle of the drug, took it home, and poured its contents into the garbage. Then, unbeknown to anyone (including my husband and kids), I replaced the pills with vitamins. I knew what I was up against,*

and I didn't want anyone else to have to lie, so it was my own little secret.

Eventually, the school told me that they wanted us to increase my son's dose. The second pill would have to be administered in the middle of the school day by the nurse. Understanding that the nurse would realize that the vitamin I had been giving my son was not Ritalin, I told the school that I would bring him the pill each day.

For the next year, I left work in the middle of the day, drove a half hour to my son's school to give him the "Ritalin" (vitamin), and then made the long trip back to work again. Finally, I told the school that my son's condition had improved and I wanted to have him reevaluated, to which they consented. I found another psychiatrist, who determined that my child no longer needed the drugs.

In response to a magazine article, which included the above story, one woman wrote, *How could she even suggest that you can cure ADHD with some vitamins?* So just to be sure that the purpose of this story is clear, the mother in the above story was not trying to *cure* ADHD with the vitamins — she was trying to prevent her son from being administered stimulant drugs, while placating the school at the same time. In fact, I know of a number of cases where teachers had falsely concluded that a student was prescribed stimulants and then noted to the parents how much improved the child's performance was. The parents, for the most part, just smiled and nodded.

Shalom,

Just to let you know, when faced with the ultimatum — Ritalin or else — I also lied to my daughter's school, telling them she was taking Ritalin while dumping it in the waste bin. At the next meeting, the teacher and the school psychologist praised my daughter's improvement, saying, "You know why she's doing better? It's because of the Ritalin!"

This happened three times. At the third meeting, when my daughter was again being sidelined by the Ritalin parade, I couldn't stand it anymore. I told them the truth: that my daughter wasn't taking Ritalin and never had.

Everyone was shocked. Including my wife. No one said a word. Not one word of apology or admittance that they were wrong. But by the next month, they were fully recovered. They put on the mask of professionalism and told me, "I'm sorry. It looks like your daughter needs Ritalin."

I sent my daughter to another school.

Nechemiah

There is no question that stimulants (or the belief that a child is taking stimulants) can have a powerful effect on children. Many parents tell me that their child is performing better in school; they even claim that the child's self-esteem is improving. But is there a cost? The use — and overuse — of stimulants has become a heated debate. While some claim that stimulants are not addictive, in reality, most are as addictive and have similar or identical properties to street drugs, like speed (methamphetamine) and cocaine.

ADDICTIVE — BUT ONLY WITHOUT A PRESCRIPTION?

While studying pharmacology during graduate school, our professor reported that the generally accepted belief among psychiatrists and manufacturers of pharmaceuticals is that when medications of an addictive nature were used therapeutically (such as codeine or morphine for surgical pain), they would not cause addiction, but that if these same drugs were used *illegally*, they could lead to drug addiction.

At the time, I was both awed and perplexed by this. I wondered: How do the mind and body know not to become dependent on these drugs just because they were accompanied by a prescription? Now I realize that the manufacturer's reassurance cannot have any basis.

Even when administered according to doctor's orders, people become addicted to prescription psychiatric drugs and pain medications all the time.

SHORT HALF-LIFE DRUGS ARE EXTREMELY ADDICTIVE

Many people receive false reassurance about stimulants. The common refrain that I hear is, "My psychiatrist told me that you cannot become addicted to Ritalin because it has a very short half-life." Meaning, its effects are *immediate*, and then it is flushed out of the system quickly. This is contrasted with longer half-life drugs, like the antidepressant Prozac, which can take a few weeks before the therapeutic effects become apparent. It takes time for Prozac to accumulate in the body, and withdrawal can be long and drawn out.

It is a misconception that the short half-life of certain stimulants prevents them from causing addiction. What it *does* mean is that many people experience withdrawal symptoms from these drugs *on a daily basis*. As many parents have reported to me, this can manifest as a rebound of hyperactivity in the afternoon, and sleeplessness at night. In fact, drugs with a short half-life can be the *most addictive*, because the user experiences withdrawal every few hours or daily, and then craves another pill.

Some psychiatrists mistakenly believe that patients will only become addicted if they *abuse* their drug and use it not as directed. While drug abuse is often blamed on the patient, the fact is that addiction commonly occurs when patients take drugs *as prescribed*.

It is well-known that we are now facing an **epidemic of prescription-drug addiction**. According to drug expert Peter Breggin, MD, "All psychiatric drugs are drugs of dependence" (i.e., addiction). Dependence means that the user experiences unpleasant effects when they stop using the drug. This invariably leads users to continue taking the drug even when they *want* to stop.

When extreme side effects and withdrawal symptoms occur, they are often attributed to the **"underlying psychiatric disorder"** rather than to the drug. Not only are psychiatric drugs acquitted from their role in triggering more severe mental "illness," but patients are often given new diagnoses, additional drugs, or higher doses when they return to their doctor complaining of new (drug-induced) symptoms.

SIDE EFFECTS

According to researchers, common side effects of stimulants include anxiety, elevated blood pressure, and seizures. So much so that the researchers have commented that "reports of adverse events in conjunction with the use of these drugs have raised concern about their safety." [103]

Additionally, every year a small percentage of stimulant users die of heart failure due to drugs taken within normal dosage range. "There is increasing concern that prescription stimulants may be associated with adverse cardiovascular events such as stroke, myocardial infarction, and sudden death."[104] Although the risk appears greater in adults, each year, stimulant-induced deaths occur in children as well.

Stimulants also frequently cause depression, insomnia, suppressed appetite, and growth suppression. "Nervousness and insomnia are the most common adverse reactions" to Ritalin, according to the manufacturers.[105] [106]

These or other unwanted symptoms are a virtual guarantee with stimulants. Although side effects may come as a surprise, they are often listed in package inserts, which are worth perusing before initiating medication.

---

103   Shaheen E. Lakhan and Annette Kirchgessner, "Prescription Stimulants in Individuals with and without Attention Deficit Hyperactivity Disorder: Misuse, Cognitive Impact, and Adverse Effects," *Brain and Behavior*, 2.5 (2012): 661–677.

104   Arthur N. Westover and Ethan A. Halm, "Do Prescription Stimulants Increase the Risk of Adverse Cardiovascular Events?: A Systematic Review," *BMC Cardiovascular Disorders*, 12 (2012): 41. PMC.

105   Eni Williams, PharmD, PhD, Ritalin Side Effects Center, Last reviewed on RxList 9/9/2016 http://www.rxlist.com/ritalin-side-effects-drug-center.htm.

106   S.M. Berman, R. Kuczenski, J.T. McCracken, London ED, "Potential Adverse Effects of Amphetamine Treatment on Brain and Behavior: A Review," *Molecular Psychiatry*, 2009;14(2):123-142. doi:10.1038/mp.2008.90.

COMMON SIDE EFFECTS

Common side effects of stimulants include addiction, depression, insomnia, suppressed appetite, growth suppression, hair loss, feminine fat distribution in boys, personality changes, bizarre behaviors, and hallucinations. It is hard to find a child who is not experiencing some of the above effects. Extreme personality changes and even suicidal ideation are so common that it is a wonder how most psychiatric drugs were granted FDA approval.

THE HAZY LINE BETWEEN THERAPEUTIC EFFECTS AND SIDE EFFECTS

According to psychiatrist Peter Breggin, MD,

Psychiatric drugs are much more dangerous than many consumers and even physicians realize... We are appalled by the widespread use of stimulants to control and suppress the behavior of children diagnosed with ADHD...

In actuality, stimulants subdue behavior by impairing mental function. They often cause the very problems they are supposed to correct... When a child seems more compliant in class or seems to attend more readily to boring, rote activities, the child is experiencing an adverse drug reaction.

ADVERSE EFFECTS OF STIMULANTS THAT ARE MISTAKEN FOR THERAPEUTIC EFFECTS*

1. Obsessive-compulsive overfocusing, inflexibility of thinking
2. Social withdrawal and isolation, reduced talking, increased solitary play

3. Behavioral suppression: compliant, apathetic, reduced curiosity and spontaneity, depressed or lethargic behavior, especially in structured environments

*Data from twenty controlled clinical trials.

When scientists experimented on lab animals by giving them stimulants, they observed a universal adverse response. This reaction occurs in humans to the same degree. Stimulants suppress behavior that is truly normal and healthy for children.

> Animals (like children) have spontaneous tendencies... to explore, to innovate, to play, to exercise, and to socialize. Dozens of studies have shown that stimulant drugs suppress all of these spontaneous tendencies, sometimes completely inhibiting them... In effect, the animals lose their "vitality" or "spirit." They become more docile and manageable. (Peter Breggin, MD)[107]

When children act spontaneously, they are called "impulsive." When they are curious, active, energetic, and want to escape the boring classroom setting, we are told they have a "brain disorder." In reality, many behaviors that are labeled as ADHD are really the normal "survival reflexes" of children.

A DIFFERENT CHILD

Many parents have told me that on stimulants, the spark of life seems to vanish from their child's eyes. Their personality can change so much that when they eventually take their child off the drugs, they tell me that they feel like they finally have their child back. Many children have also reported that despite their good grades while taking drugs, they retained *nothing* of what they learned while on medication.

107   Ibid.

Many children òn drugs are suffering. Some parents are not aware of the extent of the distress that stimulants induce in their children. People may argue that drugging children who misbehave will protect them from being treated with excessive anger and disciplinary measures, but the question is what is better for the child — spontaneous drug-free living and angry adults, or drug-induced compliance and happy adults?

For anyone who is being offered drug treatment for ADHD, I highly recommend any book by Peter R. Breggin, MD, who has been called "the conscience of modern psychiatry."

> Caution: If someone chooses to discontinue any psychiatric medication, the process must be carried out carefully to avoid dangerous withdrawal reactions. This is especially true for any child or adult who has been taking psychiatric drugs for an extended period of time. The dose should be reduced very slowly (in measures of about ten percent at a time) over a few weeks or months, under the careful supervision of a physician who understands the necessity of slowly weaning off of psychiatric drugs.

32

ADHD
SOLUTIONS

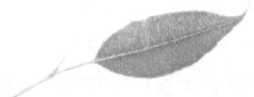

Some antidrug proponents claim that all ADHD can be treated with behavioral therapy or other forms of counseling. Although I agree with them that drugs are not the answer, and that it is highly risky to manipulate brain chemistry, some children need more than what cognitive behavioral therapy can provide because for many children, there is a physical component to their cognitive condition, which is understood better from a holistic perspective. Often, systemic issues, such as digestive and allergic problems, or exposure to external insult, can cause hyperactivity or attention problems in children.

Although herbal treatment may be appropriate for some children, I am not in favor of one-size-fits-all herbal alternatives to stimulants because these too may not address the root of the problem, and they may simply act as symptom suppressors if they work at all. Although herbal options may be safe and even beneficial, ideally, they should be used in a holistic fashion, taking into account the patient's constitution.

ALLERGIES

Some people experience strange cognitive symptoms as a result of an inflammatory reaction to food. Diet can be crucial because improper breakdown of certain foods (particularly gluten and dairy) results in the formation of intoxicating partial proteins that have a morphine-like effect on the body. This is the reason why *kids tend to be addicted to the foods that are worst for them*.

I usually recommend starting by cutting out either dairy or gluten, since they are the most common triggers. I like to eliminate one single food category at a time, because if you try to remove too many foods at once, it can become difficult, even overwhelming, and you may be left with too little food choices before getting the hang of the new diet. I find that dairy is easier to eliminate from the diet, so you may want to start with that. Stick with any dietary change for a few weeks to see if it has any effect. You can add new dietary restrictions slowly to ease the process.

ARTIFICIAL BRAIN TOXINS

Many artificial ingredients, such as monosodium glutamate (MSG), food coloring, and aspartame, act as excitotoxins in the brain. This means that they overstimulate neurons to death. Amazingly, MSG can interfere with dopamine, the neurohormone that is often implicated to be deficient in children with ADHD. When foods act like toxic drugs in the brain, it's a good idea to remove those foods, as opposed to adding other drugs to counteract the problem.[108]

VISION

Sometimes visual disturbances can manifest with symptoms that can overlap with ADHD. Vision problems that cause ADHD symptoms are rarely diagnosed by a regular optometrist and are therefore often overlooked. Anyone with reading problems, learning problems, or ADHD symptoms may have an undiagnosed vision problem. (One common example is when one eye is dominant and the other is lazy but would never receive a typical diagnosis of "lazy eye.")

---

108   Russell L. Blaylock, MD, *Excitotoxins: The Taste that Kills*, 1997, Health Press.

It is a good idea to search for an ADHD vision therapist in your area. A vision therapist will take into account eye problems that do not manifest as typical vision problems. They will then create a customized treatment plan, which may include an assortment of eye exercises. Sometimes they give the child a specially designed computer-exercise program. Many people have reported great improvement in their learning, reading, and concentration after receiving vision therapy.

Recently, I have seen advertisements in Israel for a computer game that was apparently developed by NASA scientists, with the promise of treating ADHD. With the possible exception of the computer eye-exercise programs to improve vision mentioned above, it is my belief that computer games only make children's brains less effective, and I am particularly wary of anything coming out of NASA.

HEAVY METALS

A huge factor that contributes to many health problems, but especially neurodevelopmental delays like learning disabilities, ADHD, speech problems, and even extreme cognitive impairment in today's children is *an overload of poisons, particularly from heavy metals* (such as mercury, aluminum, and lead). Where is the heavy metal coming from? Mercury can be found in silver (amalgam) cavity fillings, tuna and other fish, but especially in some vaccines (flu, DTaP). Aluminum is found in foil bakeware, as well as antiperspirants and other cosmetics, and in vaccines.

Heavy Metal Detoxification

To remove heavy metals from the body, one may try home remedies such as activated charcoal, bentonite clay, high doses of vitamin C, B vitamins, as well as herbs such as chlorella and cilantro and even garlic, which have reportedly been effective. They should be used under the guidance of a health practitioner experienced in detoxification.

Heavy metal toxicologists make use of pharmaceutical drugs to detoxify children and adults who have been poisoned by heavy metals. They are known as "chelating agents." This process has returned some children with severe neurodevelopmental delays to near normalcy. The most common chelators are EDTA and DMSA. Recently, another chelator, called transdermal DMPS, has joined the ranks and may be a good option for children since it is applied via a patch rather than injection or pills. Mineral supplements must be taken when using chelating agents. The process should be supervised by a knowledgeable (preferably holistically minded) heavy metal toxicologist.

INTESTINAL PARASITES

Sometimes intestinal parasites (most commonly in the form of pinworm) can cause behavioral and even personality changes. Many parents have reported as much to me. Parasitic infection can be very chronic and yet may often go undiagnosed. For some children, ADHD simply vanishes when they receive effective treatment to eliminate parasites.

BIRTH TRAUMA

Another important factor that can contribute to brain development issues is birth trauma, such as a cesarean, a prolonged or difficult birth, or diminished blood flow to the baby (causing reduced oxygen to the brain) during birth. Recent evidence suggests that ultrasound and Doppler, including fetal monitoring during labor, may damage the brains of infants. Sometimes it is possible to heal from this sort of trauma. Craniosacral therapy, "One Brain" therapy, health kinesiology, 3-D therapy, or treatments to integrate infantile reflexes may be beneficial.

SOCIAL TROUBLE

Some children act out because they are being bullied or mistreated, or have experienced some kind of abuse or trauma. Also, children of all ages are extraordinarily sensitive to disharmony in the home. Children often act out unhappiness with misbehavior. When these children misbehave, they are crying for help! How many abused children have been drugged into submission for behavioral problems, taking away their ability to express their distress and get real help?

Play therapy or drawing analysis can be an effective way to get into a child's world and discover what he is experiencing. EMDR (eye movement desensitization and reprocessing) therapy is a powerful new tool to help recover from trauma, but is more appropriate for older children or adults.

GENERAL MODALITIES FOR ADHD

There is no single remedy or protocol that will work for every child. Some will benefit from vitamins or calming mineral supplements such as calcium, magnesium and zinc, or a B complex. Some will respond well to omega-3 fish oil. Acupuncture and herbal medicine can do wonders for some children, while others will make great strides with craniosacral therapy. Some respond to homeopathy, while others benefit from vision therapy. Exercise and martial arts have been very helpful for many children. Don't get overwhelmed by this list! Try one thing at a time, without holding your breath for instant results. Change does not happen overnight. The main thing is to choose treatments that are safe with little or no potential to cause serious harm or dangerous side effects.

33

THE MIND

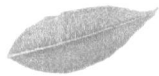

In recent times, modern society has become aware of the fact that the mind has a major impact on our health. It can be compared to Columbus discovering America; he is given a lot of credit for finding this unexplored region, yet the fact that the land was already teeming with natives was not really relevant to anyone. It has been long understood by most traditional medical systems that the mind plays a crucial role in health.

When one is told that the ailment he is suffering from is "psychosomatic" (meaning, the bodily symptoms are caused by the mind), he will probably leave the doctor feeling a bit indignant. He may feel that his doctor believes that there isn't really anything wrong at all, and that he is imagining his pain. This is a valid concern, as most doctors use the term "psychosomatic" with the implication that the disease does *not* exist outside of the patient's mind.

However, many conclude erroneously that an illness rooted in the mind isn't real. There is such a negative impression of diseases with any emotional component that I have to be careful in my clinic not to make such "accusations." Patients get defensive.

Chinese medicine (which is about two thousand years old) lists different causes of diseases. These include, diet, lifestyle, the external environment, infection, and the emotions. Illnesses caused by the emotions are not imaginary; the mind is capable of producing a *real* pathological process in the body. A malady caused by the emotions is not in your head at all, it's exactly where you feel it. However, the *source* of the problem is the mind.

DIGESTION

A good example of the mind-body connection in the generation of disease can be seen in digestive ailments, such as irritable bowel syndrome (IBS) or Crohn's disease. Stress and tension cause a real chemical response in the body. Under stress, the human body releases catecholamine, the stress hormone. This produces what is known as the fight-or-flight response.

When catecholamine is released, the pupils dilate, the heart rate increases, the blood pressure rises, and circulation is shunted away from all organs that are not necessary in an emergency, such as the digestive system. People should not spend more than about 2 percent of their lives in this state.

If someone experiences a lot of stress, their digestive system is constantly being shut down, leaving them with chronic digestive disturbance. To effect a cure for stress-induced digestive trouble, the mental aspect must be addressed. Not all digestive problems are rooted in the emotions, but if they are, the illness is just as real.

PAIN

A few years ago, a woman came to me suffering from fibromyalgia (an ailment associated with severe chronic pain). Acupuncture treatments produced good results, but at a certain point, we reached a plateau where the treatments would go no further. Knowing that fibromyalgia is often rooted in the emotions, I tried to present this to my patient. Her response was defensive, and I was forced to put the mental aspects aside.

She felt that I was assuming that her illness was imagined. This could not have been further from the truth; I could see with my own eyes that blood had become stuck in certain parts of her body, and that the muscles were in spasm, producing pain. The illness was real, but the mental connection could not be ignored. By accepting the reality that certain diseases are rooted in the mind, the issue can be addressed at its source and resolved on all levels.

Pain is a result of stagnation, meaning that there is an interruption in the normal flow of blood, fluids, or physical energy (*chi* or *qi*) in the body. There are various causes of stagnation. It may be environmental (as in joint pain experienced in humid or cold weather), it may be structural, or there may be some other underlying illness that is causing the blockage.

The other possibility is that because of stress, anger, worry, fear, or another negative emotion, the mind has shut down the body's normal flow, causing pain. In Chinese medicine, this is considered just as valid and common a diagnosis as the previous ones.

PHYSICAL CAUSES

During the past few decades, the mood-controlling hormones of the brain have received a lot of attention. There are many known physical causes for mental imbalances. For example, in Chinese medicine, one possible cause of depression is blood deficiency, which is comparable, though not identical, to anemia (low iron). This can be understood as the brain not receiving proper nourishment due to lack of blood. A poorly nourished brain is likely to malfunction and cause mood changes. Note: Many people have reported to me that B vitamins greatly improved their moods.

Poor eating habits (white flour, sugar, etc.) can lead to malnourishment, which commonly has a bad effect on the mind. Lack of sleep or exercise can also cause our minds to play tricks on us. In these situations, the mental disorder is rooted in a physical deficit. If something in the body is lacking, the only way to solve the problem at its root is to correct the deficiency in the body.

TRAUMATIC EVENTS

By far the most painful situation I have seen is in people who are suffering because of some form of trauma. For some, it may have been a miserable life situation in the past or present, a sort of chronic trauma. For others, it was the untimely or unexpected death of a close relative. Some are suffering from serious relationship problems or a history of abuse, or they may simply have gone through a very stressful situation and are feeling depressed and out of sorts.

Often, these people are labeled with a psychiatric disorder, such as depression, anxiety, or bipolar disorder, and are given a prescription to go with the diagnosis.

Knowing that traumatic events have a tendency to cause anxiety or depression, can we truly call something a mental illness if it is a person's reaction to a painful life experience?

Even if mental illness would be the appropriate label, is the appropriate response to mask the symptoms with psychiatric drugs? It seems obvious that the traumatic experience must be worked through, and not ignored or even buried with drugs. In many cases, exercise and therapy can do more than drugs!

In my clinical experience, I have observed that very often the person is still suffering from some form of abuse or post trauma. All this is overlooked when psychiatric diseases and medication become the focal point. The focus on the person's current symptoms to the exclusion of their life history or current circumstances can distract those trying to assist from the real source of suffering.

THE SOURPUSS

While the source of depression may often be chemical, physical, or traumatic, there is another aspect that deserves more attention. That is our own ability to control our thoughts and feelings. The modern emphasis on brain chemistry controlling our moods has led people to the mistaken conclusion that our emotional state is generally out of our hands.

While there certainly are situations of mental illness where one loses control over their emotions and thoughts (ranging from postpartum depression to schizophrenia), there are occasions where our belief that we have no control only causes the situation to deteriorate. The truth is that we have control over nothing in this world *except* our thoughts. In many situations, our thought patterns alone will ultimately have the greatest influence over our mood.

A common scenario occurs in people who are frequently depressed due to an overly negative view on life. They see only the bad in every situation and cannot enjoy any part of life because they are drowning in negativity and self-pity. These people do not make good company. In this situation, a person can transform their existence by changing their focus and learning to appreciate the good that has been bestowed upon them.

Positivity Exercise[109]

> *Imagine you are witness to someone who is standing in the window of a skyscraper, about to jump.*
>
> *"Wait!" you call to him.*
>
> *"Leave me alone unless you want to come with me!"*
>
> *"Wait!" you repeat. "What if you'd been blind your whole life, and just now, as you're about to jump, your vision came back... Would you still jump?"*
>
> *The man turns to you and backs away a bit from ledge. "No, I'd want to go and see the world..."*
>
> *"Well, you can see! Are you sure you don't want to go see the world?"*

No matter how miserable a person's life may be, there is always something to appreciate. Sometimes it can take a bit of digging, but it is well worth the effort.

---

109   As heard from Rabbi Aharon Goldman.

APPENDIX A:
NATURAL
HOME REMEDIES

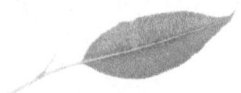

As a practitioner of Chinese medicine, I have seen how effective natural remedies can be. While Chinese herbs are especially useful for chronic problems like asthma, chronic coughs, seasonal allergies, arthritis, or women's health, for everyday use, they have some drawbacks. You have to get the prescription from a knowledgeable herbalist, since nearly every formula is custom-tailored for the individual situation, so you can't keep them handy in your medicine cabinet to pull out as needed.

BENEFITS OF NATURAL HOME REMEDIES

- They're usually inexpensive.
- You don't need a prescription.
- You can buy many of them anywhere.
- You can keep them on hand to use as needed.
- Many have multiple uses.
- They're safe and have minimal side effects.
- You may have some of them in your house already.
- When they work, they work well.

In my experience, many simple home remedies can be more effective than over-the-counter options with too many ingredients. For example, bacitracin can produce disappointing results. I have found this substance to be about as effective as Vaseline in preventing or healing wound infections. (Don't ever put Vaseline on an open wound.) In this appendix you will find a lot of far more effective options.

Some remedies are great for one issue, but useless for another. Some remedies take time, while with others you'll see results right away. I am only sharing remedies that I have seen be effective for my patients. Nothing works for everyone, but I have chosen these remedies based on their ability to produce positive results time after time. The remedies are listed in no particular order.

Hydrogen Peroxide

Where to get it

In Israel (where I live), you can only get hydrogen peroxide at a pharmacy. It comes in tiny bottles of 100 ml, which is about 3.3 oz. This is mightily frustrating, since it's such a useful substance. For the same price, you can get *ten times* this amount in the US, where you'll find it in most grocery stores and pharmacies.

Uses

Whenever my sister-in-law calls me up for advice for any health problem, I tell her, "Try hydrogen peroxide!" It's become a bit of a running joke between us. But the truth is that hydrogen peroxide has many uses. It is known as a wound disinfectant, and it is incredible for that.

Wounds: Pour some hydrogen peroxide on clean, dry wounds. For more serious, stubborn, or inflamed wounds, soak a cotton ball in hydrogen peroxide, then place it on the wound for as long as possible. Do this a few times a day. Alternatively, wrap gauze around the soaked cotton ball and leave it in place for a few hours or overnight.

The reason hydrogen peroxide works even when antibiotic ointments have no effect is probably because of its ability to break up hard scabs, penetrate the infected wound beneath, and then kill the bacteria. It does not damage healthy tissue while it destroys dead or diseased tissue. Hydrogen peroxide can burn a bit when you put it on, but it's very effective.

Many infectious bacteria are anaerobic. This means that they survive better without oxygen. Oxygen actually kills these unhealthy bacteria. This is why it's important to avoid Band-Aids, and expose wounds to open air to promote healing.

Band-Aids work great for boo-boos! I tell my kids to put the Band-Aid anywhere except the boo-boo. My kids happily accept them as a consolation prize.

Hydrogen peroxide is H_2O_2, which is like water with an extra oxygen atom. The oxygen bombards anaerobic bacteria and kills them quickly. Unlike antibiotics, bacteria do not seem capable of developing resistance to this substance.

Ear-piercing infections: Replace whatever earrings you've been wearing with solid gold earrings to prevent the hole from closing, and apply hydrogen peroxide to the infected earlobe twice a day. Interestingly, gold has antimicrobial effects as well, which is why you should wear gold earrings if your lobes get infected.

Gargle: According to the bottle, you can use hydrogen peroxide as an "oral debriding agent." This means it helps clean your teeth. But you can also use it to clean your tonsils, which may clear an impending strep throat. Gargle with hydrogen peroxide a few times a day at the first sign of a sore throat.

Foot fungus: Spray hydrogen peroxide directly onto your feet, or use as a foot soak. This can be as effective as any antifungal spray, probably even better. For toenail fungus, submerge your nails and soak for five to fifteen minutes daily. Beware that hydrogen peroxide will destroy leather shoes.

Tip: You can use your Crocs to soak your feet.

Preventing toe infection: Although I have successfully treated toe infections with Chinese herbs, preventing infection is preferable. Toe infections are common on the big toe, and are often the result of cutting the nails a bit too close to the corner of the nail bed. To prevent this, spray hydrogen peroxide on your toenails every time you cut them.

Household cleaner: Literally a "home" remedy. Kills mold and can be great for cleaning damp hard surfaces found in bathrooms and kitchens. Hydrogen peroxide will not work as well as bleach on mildew stains, but it's really fun to watch it bubble when you spray it on organic matter. This is a chemical reaction that frees the oxygen and leaves just water behind.

Stain remover: Especially good for blood stains. All laundry chemicals with names like "oxy" or "oxygen" rely on the same chemical reaction that hydrogen peroxide produces.

Iodine

Where to get it

You can find iodine for external use at most pharmacies. If you want to use it as a gargle, I recommend an edible form, like Lugol's Solution, which is a quality yet affordable option. If your pharmacy doesn't have Lugol's, you may have to order it online.

Uses

Iodine is a broad-spectrum antimicrobial that can kill fungus, bacteria, and viruses. In my experience, it works *best* for fungus. You can try it as a gargle for sore throat as well, but only use an edible form of iodine for gargling. It will feel sore at first, but better soon after that if it's working for you.

Fungus: Iodine is great for any area that gets damp, sweaty, and itchy, such as jock itch and underarm rash. Test iodine on a small area of your skin to make sure that it doesn't irritate you. Apply any type of iodine for itchy rashes; experiment with liquids or ointments. It may burn a little at first, but it should calm down after a few minutes. If it's working for you, then you should feel immediate relief. Warning: Iodine is brown, and though it is washable, it will temporarily stain your clothing yellow.

Diaper rash: Diaper rash can quickly become infected. Apply iodine ointment to prevent or cure early signs of infection. Also change diapers frequently, or let your child spend some time diaperless, since exposure to air prevents infection and promotes healing. (I would put "air" on my list of top remedies too, but I think most people already know how to use it.)

Eczema: According to Medical News Today,

> Atopic eczema is on the increase, and while we don't know
> what causes it or how to cure it, we do know that one of the
> triggers is the yeast M. sympodialis, one of the most com-
> mon skin yeasts in both healthy people and those suffering
> from eczema. Usually our skin barrier stops the yeast from
> causing infection, but in people with eczema, the barrier is
> often more fragile or even broken, so it allows the yeast to
> cause infection and make the condition worse.[110]

Many mothers have reported to me that iodine ointment gave
their infants and children much relief, even for extremely irritated
eczema. Eczema may be caused or exacerbated by microbial infection.
Since iodine is a broad-spectrum antimicrobial, this may be why it
works for eczema. Again, it may cause some initial irritation, but
after a few minutes there should be relief. With persistent use, some
may find that the eczema completely clears. Only use long-term if
you see good results.

Warts: One book that I read on home remedies recommended iodine
ointment for treating warts. Don't bother using it for this problem
because it's not nearly as effective as something everybody should have
in their pantry:

Apple Cider Vinegar

Where to get it

You can get it at any grocery store. Look for one that is preservative
free. (I find it absurd that some vinegars have preservatives when vinegar *is* a preservative!) Apple cider vinegar has been used to cure nearly
every disease under the sun. The following list is not extensive, but
merely based on successes that I can verify because I have personally
witnessed them.

---

110   Paddock C, "Eczema Yeast Can Be Killed Off, Raising Hope of New Treatments," Medical
      News Today, November 2011.

Uses

Warts:

> *When I was a kid, I had a wart burned off my finger by a dermatologist. Apparently, some of it was left behind, because it started to come back again. More burning. Twenty-five years later, I still have scars to show for it. I wish I had known about apple cider vinegar. I tried iodine on my daughter's wart. It didn't seem to do much. Then I tried apple cider vinegar. It caused a small wart on my daughter's finger to simply vanish. No scar.*
>
> *Then we tried it on a stubborn and painful plantar wart (on the bottom of the foot) on one of my other kids. We kept it up for weeks. I made the method simpler by dripping a bit of vinegar on a Band-Aid. The wart started to blacken, which I know is a good sign. We took a break over Pesach, thinking that the wart was already on the way out. It came back with a vengeance, and after Pesach we had to start over. This time, we were really persistent and applied a vinegar Band-Aid morning and evening. It took a few weeks, but the stubborn wart finally fell out. I have heard that plantar warts can last for years and have a tendency to spread. Apple cider vinegar is officially my new best friend!*

Mosquito bites: Try swiping a bit of apple cider vinegar over an itchy mosquito bite. When it works, it provides instant relief.

Eczema: Apple cider vinegar, once again upstaging iodine, appears to be one of the most effective home remedies for curing eczema. Scratch that. It's more effective than prescription treatments as well! Use a cotton ball and apply vinegar directly over all affected areas once daily. If the area is raw or was recently scratched, it may sting a little, but the feeling will disappear as soon as the vinegar dries. While many recommend organic, I have seen good results with non-organic as well.

Multi-use apple cider vinegar beverage: Add a tablespoon of vinegar to a cup of water and drink before meals to prevent acid reflux and treat insulin sensitivity,[111] or any time to prevent dehydration,[112] improve digestion, and cleanse the bowels. If you love it, you can even try your luck against a common cold, strep throat, or flu.[113]

Household cleaner: Put a combo of vinegar and water (at about a one to eight ratio, but it's not an exact science) in a spray bottle to create a nontoxic cleaner that is even effective against household bacteria. You can add a few drops of essential oil for aroma.

Baking Soda

Where to get it

Anywhere.

Uses

Foot deodorant: Pour baking soda into your shoes if you have smelly feet. Though you may be tempted, be careful about using baking soda on inflamed rashes; I have seen it aggravate problems like diaper rash or jock itch.

Thrush: Dip a wet cotton swab into baking soda and apply directly to the spots in the baby's mouth. For thrush on mom, try **gentian violet**.

Yeast infection: Add half to one cup of baking soda to a warm bath. Stir it well and soak for about twenty minutes. Rinse afterward.

Baking soda beverage: Add a few pinches or up to two teaspoons to water to prevent dehydration and treat acid reflux or indigestion. Some people love baking soda in their water, some find it nauseating. Only use it if you find it palatable.

Putting out fires: Not exactly a medicinal use, but potentially life-saving, so worth mentioning. Keep a container of baking soda on hand in your kitchen in case of emergency.

---

111   Johnston CS, Kim C, and Buller AJ, "Vinegar Improves Insulin Sensitivity to a High-Carbohydrate Meal in Subjects with Insulin Resistance or Type 2 Diabetes," *Diabetes Care*, 2004 Jan; 27(1): 281–282 https://doi.org/10.2337/diacare.27.1.281, ADA.

112   According to *Rashi* on *Megillas Rus* 2:14.

113   Axe J, "20 Unique Apple Cider Vinegar Uses and Benefits," draxe.com/apple-cider-vinegar-uses/.

On Chanukah about twelve years ago, there was a mishap at my in-laws' house when a frying pan of latkes caught fire. It was suddenly huge and terrifying! My husband immediately swung into action and started throwing open the cabinets in search of baking soda. He found baking powder in a Pesach (Passover) cabinet and tossed it over the fire, smothering the flames. My mother-in-law forgave him for opening the Pesach cabinets in the middle of the year, and we all commended him on his quick thinking — it wasn't baking soda, but it did the job.

Household cleaning:

- **Frying pans:** For stuck-on grease, sprinkle with baking soda while the pan is still hot (you can even leave a small flame on), then add water. As it comes to a boil, it will lift most of the burned matter right off the surface of the pan. Leave for twenty minutes before attempting to scrub it.
- **General cleaning:** Put baking soda in a spice container and sprinkle it over hard surfaces (like sinks, counters, tubs, and tiles) and scrub.
- **Drain cleaner:** Pour up to a cup of baking soda and a cup of vinegar down sink drain, let it bubble for about fifteen minutes, then wash it down with hot or boiling water.
- **Dishwasher:** Add to your dishwasher to degrease.
- **Laundry:** Add up to a cup of baking soda to the detergent section of your washing machine. Baking soda acts as a deodorizer and a fabric softener.
  Note: Chemical fabric softeners leave harmful residue on laundry that can irritate sensitive skin. If you dry dishes with dish towels that were washed with fabric softener, you are then eating fabric softener, which is a very bad idea. *Towels are actually more absorbent without chemical fabric softeners.*
  About thirteen years ago, I discovered that fabric softener creates a coating on the dryer's lint trap that prevents air from

passing through and shortens the lifespan of the dryer. The way to test this is by rinsing the lint trap with cold water — if it's coated with residue, the water will bead on the surface instead of passing through. For all these reasons, I haven't used fabric softener since then, but I do use baking soda in my laundry nearly every day.

Tea Tree Oil

Where to get it

In Israel, they sell it in pharmacies. If you can't find it in your local pharmacy, try a health-food store, or buy it online. With tea tree oil, you get what you pay for; look for the highest-grade product. It should be 100 percent pure, with no additives or other oils. The percent of the active ingredient Terpinen will determine its potency. Terpinen content can range from 10 to 45 percent. Beware that although higher potencies are more powerful, if you have sensitive skin, the higher levels of Terpinen may irritate your skin. Quality tea tree should be sold in a dark brown glass bottle, and stored away from light and air.

Tea tree oil is strong stuff. Some people like to use it straight up, but because of its strength, many people need to mix a few drops of it into a carrier oil, like a spoon of olive oil, or a bit of water. Try it both ways to see which feels better. **Always test tea tree oil on a small area of the skin first to make sure it doesn't cause irritation.**

Uses

Natural deodorant: Tea tree oil's antimicrobial qualities can kill the bacteria that cause underarm odor. You can rub a drop under each arm instead of deodorant. I think it has a lovely smell, but some people think it smells like Pine Sol.

Mosquito repellent: Tea tree oil was recommended to me by a colleague over ten years ago to relieve itching from mosquito bites. While attempting to use it for this purpose, I accidentally discovered that it's also a great mosquito repellent. **Citronella** essential oil is also a good mosquito repellent (but not useful enough to warrant its own subtopic. Sorry, citronella).

Acne: A safe and effective alternative to harsh cleaners. Use a Q-tip to dab a drop onto each pimple and leave on for a few hours or overnight. For Terpinen content higher than fifteen percent, test your sensitivity and dilute if necessary with a small amount of water before applying.

To make a gentle acne face wash, mix five drops of tea tree oil with two teaspoons of raw honey. Rub the mixture on your face, leave on for one to five minutes, and then rinse it off.[114]

Lice repellent: Mix twenty drops into a bottle of shampoo to create a lice-repellent effect. Don't expect this to completely resolve a current lice infestation, only to keep future invasions at bay. **Lavender** essential oil may also be used for this purpose.

Gargle: Mix a drop or two with a little water as a mouthwash or gargle. It will freshen your breath and may also keep tonsillitis at bay.

Yeast infection: Mix a few drops into water and wash the area with it, or soak in a shallow bath. It may sting a little, but it should bring immediate relief after that.

Toenail fungus: In my practice I have seen thousands of toes, and it is rare to find anyone over the age of thirty who does not have some toenail fungus. Toenail fungus is not a popular topic of conversation, so most people have no idea that they're in good company.

I have not seen tea tree oil work for toenail fungus, but perhaps it may work better if combined 50:50 with oregano oil. Consider combining with hydrogen peroxide treatment (see above).

Antifungal: In addition to being antibacterial, tea tree oil can be used on itchy skin rashes that are caused by fungus. This will be a better option for you than iodine if you're wearing a white shirt. Discontinue if you notice ongoing irritation, or no relief.

Colloidal Silver

Where to get it

In Israel, where I live, colloidal silver can be hard to find. It's a really effective natural, broad-spectrum antimicrobial, and I can't help but wonder why the Ministry of Health doesn't like it. I recently found a supplier locally

---

114 Axe J, "Top 10 Tea Tree Oil Uses and Benefits," draxe.com/tea-tree-oil-uses-benefits/.

and have begun testing its uses. In the US, it is much more readily available, and can be purchased online or at health-food stores. Quality can vary greatly, so look for products that have received a lot of positive reviews.

Uses

Colloidal silver is made up of tiny nanoparticles of pure metallic silver, suspended in water. The silver is very dilute and is measured in parts per million (PPM). The smaller the silver particles in the solution, the more medicinal power the product will have. The microparticles of silver block bacterial respiration and also prevent microbial reproduction. Laboratory experiments have shown that at least 650 microbes were destroyed upon exposure to colloidal silver.

Silver is a broad-spectrum antimicrobial. It does not damage overall health like antibiotics. So far, evidence seems to indicate that bacteria cannot develop resistance to silver like they do to antibiotics, in which case colloidal silver may be a viable solution to the ever-increasing number of antibiotic-resistant strains of bacteria. Silver is highly effective for many infections, and is great for both external and internal use.

External application: Colloidal silver can be sprayed on skin infections, eye infections, or, for ear infections, dropped into the ear and left for five minutes (hydrogen peroxide may also be used for earache). It can be used as a nasal spray for sinus infection. It can be gargled and then swallowed for sore throat and tonsillitis. Its uses for external infection are pretty much limitless. It can be used for fungus (such as thrush) and viruses (such as shingles) as well. It may even be effective in skin conditions that are not clearly rooted in infection, such as psoriasis or eczema. In most cases, when it is used externally, silver should also be taken internally for maximum effect.

Internal use: Colloidal silver can be taken internally for many kinds of infections, including colds and flu, bronchitis or pneumonia (even cases that are resistant to antibiotic treatment), strep throat, ear infection, urinary tract infection, all kinds of viral infections, and fungal/yeast infections. It may be beneficial for certain chronic diseases as well, and is worth investigating for any health problem that is not responding to other treatments.

Nebulizer: One teaspoon of colloidal silver can be added to a nebulizer and used three times a day, with the vapors inhaled for ten to fifteen minutes to treat any kind of chest infection or inflammation.

Vitamin C

In 1975, Australian physician Archie Kalokerinos, MD, was called upon to care for the very sick Aborigine population (the Australian natives). Of particular concern was the incredibly high death rate among Aborigine children. Astoundingly, one in every two Aborigine babies was dying (hence, the title of his book, *Every Second Child*).[115]

He discovered two important things, the first of which was that children were dying after receiving vaccinations. Many of the children were already sick before vaccination, which led to his second discovery, that the children were extremely malnourished; in particular, they were deficient in vitamin C. The vitamin C deficiency caused them to be incredibly susceptible to illness. Since vitamin C is depleted by illness or vaccination (among other stressors), the vaccines pushed them over the brink and ultimately caused their demise.

He realized that by supplementing these children with modest doses of vitamin C, he could prevent most, if not all, deaths. He continued to supplement and vaccinate, but later realized that the vaccines were not helping to prevent death (since they were causing death), and he eventually recommended against vaccination altogether. To his frustration, Dr. Kalokerinos's discoveries about the deadly potential of vitamin C deficiency and vaccine-related scurvy deaths went completely unheeded by medical authorities worldwide. This was despite the fact that simply supplementing with vitamin C has the potential to prevent disease and death, particularly in impoverished, malnourished populations.

Vitamin C deficiency is common among people across the world, not only those under primitive conditions. People who eat few fruits and vegetables are likely to be deficient. If the deficiency is severe enough, it can cause scurvy, a potentially deadly condition. To prevent scurvy, European sailors ate fermented cabbage (sauerkraut), and Chinese

---

115   Archie Kalokerinos, MD, *Every Second Child*, 1974.

sailors ate bean sprouts throughout their long sea journeys. The vitamin C content in these vegetables actually increases during the fermentation/sprouting process. These dietary methods were highly effective in preventing scurvy deaths among sailors.

Most people today are aware of the importance of vitamin C. Some, however, are not aware of how little of the vitamin is actually present in most fruits and vegetables. We have also been sorely misinformed about how much is needed on a daily basis. The US Recommended Daily Allowance (RDA) of vitamin C is 60 mg, which has caused much suspicion among educated consumers, since this amount is so minute. Most people probably need about ten times this dose. Aware of the inadequacy of the Recommended Daily Allowance, most vitamin manufacturers offer supplements with a minimum of 250 mg per dose, which is over four times the RDA suggestion.

For example, when orange juice containers claim that one cup of juice contains 100 percent daily value of vitamin C, this is highly misleading. Firstly, most orange juice contains *no* vitamin C, because the juice is pasteurized and heat destroys vitamin C. Exposure to air over time also causes vitamin C content to diminish, so bottled juices are not likely to contain much vitamin C at all. Secondly, even if there were 60 mg in every cup of juice, this is a dangerously inadequate dose, approaching scurvy levels. Since soil quality today is poor in many places, many fresh fruits and vegetables contain far less vitamin C than expected. So unless you have a fresh daily supply of high-quality organically-grown fruits and vegetables, it is recommended that you take a vitamin C supplement every day.

The best way to take vitamin C is in small doses (250 mg) throughout the day, because the body uses it quickly but cannot store it, so excess will be wasted. Just like water, you can't drink your day's supply first thing in the morning and hope you won't need another drink for the rest of the day (unless you're a camel). Fat-soluble vitamins, like A, D, E, and K can be stored longer in the body and don't necessarily need to be taken daily. If you are pressed for time, or if the thought of taking supplements throughout the day sounds daunting, especially if you are not in the midst of fighting an illness, you can take 250 mg to 1000 mg of vitamin C once a day.

Vitamin C comes in many forms. For children, ascorbic acid is usually preferred, because it's sour and can be sweetened to create a pleasant taste. Other versions, like sodium or calcium ascorbate can be great in pill form, but they are bitter and unpalatable for children. In our home, we dissolve ascorbic-acid powder in water and add fruit juice concentrate for the kids. The adults mix it with plain water or seltzer. To boost immune function, the best way is to take small amounts throughout the day. Large doses can have a laxative effect, which may be beneficial for those in need of a laxative.

The laxative effect of vitamin C is the reason why there is no concern about overdosing. Once your body has absorbed all it can, the rest will be eliminated through the bowels. The one exception to the safety of large doses of vitamin is during pregnancy. Doses of 6,000 mg per day in early pregnancy can be abortifacient (induce miscarriage) for some women. Therefore, pregnant women should take no more than 2,000 mg of vitamin C a day. The dose that causes diarrhea is known as "bowel tolerance"; it is considered beneficial for individuals to figure out how many milligrams cause this effect and then take a bit less than that each day.

In addition to supporting the immune system, vitamin C is also a detoxifier and nature's antibiotic. It has been used to remove deadly poisons, such as after exposure to toxic heavy metals or pesticides. The following important and lifesaving medical breakthrough has sadly been largely forgotten by the world: In 1949, Dr. Fred Klenner reported successful treatment against polio, diphtheria, herpes zoster, herpes simplex, chicken pox, influenza, measles, mumps, and viral pneumonia with injections of large doses of vitamin C. He wrote, "The results of using vitamin C as the antibiotic, which we have reported in *Virus Diseases*, may seem fantastic."

I will point out that antibiotics kill bacteria and are ineffective against viruses, but Dr. Klenner's experience with vitamin C shows that its effects are far more broad than antibiotics, having the ability to treat viruses as well. Despite the existence of antivirals, modern medicine has no truly effective treatment for viruses, since antivirals are not very effective. One might expect the medical world to jump on an effective and inexpensive option like vitamin C. Instead, the medical establishment recommends doses that are too small to have any curative effect, offering just enough to keep healthy people from dying of scurvy.

APPENDIX B: SOLUTIONS FOR BREECH BABIES

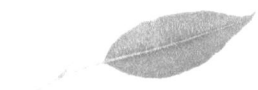

Before ultrasound became standard, many healthcare providers determined fetal position with their hands. Though there are still medical practitioners capable of performing this exam, it is increasingly becoming a lost art. Whichever method is used to determine fetal position, it is helpful to check that the baby is in a head-down position.

Since cesareans are unjustifiably favored, another lost art is the natural delivery of breech babies. It can be hard to find a doctor or midwife who is willing or able to do so. Therefore, head down is the ideal position for a natural delivery. I recommend that women get checked for fetal position between thirty and thirty-four weeks. At this point, there is still room for the baby to turn. Earlier, there is too much room, so the baby can turn back. Later on, there may not be enough room for the baby to turn using gentle methods.

There are a number of ways to turn the fetus head down.

One highly effective and safe option is **acupuncture and Chinese moxibustion** (specifically the bladder points on the pinky toes — UB 67). Studies show that using moxibustion at the right time can help turn the baby to a head-down position around eighty percent of the time. I have personally seen this method work for many women.

Deep relaxation or hypnosis for expectant mothers can also help make the womb more pliant and flexible so that there is room for the baby to move into the right position easily.

Some women try putting **ice packs** near the ribs and **warmth** on the lower abdomen, which may encourage the baby to move its head down.

Shining **light** or playing **music** at the lower abdomen, to attract the baby to turn down, is also worth trying.

Some try a **tilt board**, with the feet up and the head down, or headstands in a swimming pool. This should not be attempted if the baby may have already turned, because it may cause the head to turn back up!

Women often feel the baby turn while using these techniques. When these methods work, the results can be immediate.

External cephalic version (ECV), manually turning the baby, is the last resort and ideally should not be used before thirty-seven weeks. It is not risk-free and may pull the umbilical cord into a position that is not good for the fetus, or worse. This may be why many babies turn back to breech positions after external version — to release the umbilical cord from an awkward position. Though external version is a last resort, it is still safer for the mother and baby than a cesarean, and it may even be used during labor. Although thirty to thirty-four weeks is the ideal time for all techniques except ECV, all of the above methods (and more) should be tried up until the birth.

INDEX

ABOUT THE AUTHOR

Yael Tusk, MSc, is trained in designing and evaluating scientific studies, and specializes in researching and debunking scientific myths. In addition to researching and writing, she is a practitioner of Chinese medicine in Jerusalem, where she treats both adults and children.

More information about the services she offers at the Center for Natural Medicine can be found at www.yaeltusk.com.

ABOUT THE CENTER FOR NATURAL MEDICINE

Jerusalem's Center for Natural Medicine provides treatment with Traditional Chinese Medicine, including acupuncture, herbal medicine, and general health counseling for both local patients and via phone consultation for international clientele. For over a decade, Yael Tusk, MSOM, has been treating adults and children for ailments ranging from the common cold and colic to depression and infertility.

Check out Yaeltusk.com for more information about the clinic. You can also sign up for the informative monthly *Natural Health Update* through the website.

www.ingramcontent.com/pod-product-compliance
Lightning Source LLC
Chambersburg PA
CBHW051343280526
45784CB00007B/2797